Letting in
the

WILD EDGES

Glennie Kindred

PERMANENT PUBLICATIONS

Published by
Permanent Publications
Hyden House Ltd
The Sustainability Centre
East Meon
Hampshire GU32 1HR
England
Tel: 01730 823 311
Fax: 01730 823 322
Overseas: (international code +44 - 1730)
Email: enquiries@permaculture.co.uk
Web: www.permaculture.co.uk

Distributed in the USA by
Chelsea Green Publishing Company, PO Box 428, White River Junction, VT 05001
www.chelseagreen.com

Designed by Tim Harland

Cover design by Sarah Howerd, www.sideways14.co.uk

Printed in the UK by Cambrian Printers, Aberystwyth

All paper from FSC certified mixed sources

The Forest Stewardship Council (FSC) is a non-profit international organisation
established to promote the responsible management of the world's forests. Products
carrying the FSC label are independently certified to assure consumers that they come
from forests that are managed to meet the social, economic and ecological needs of
present and future generations.

British Library Cataloguing-in-Publication Data
A catalogue record for this book is available from the British Library
ISBN 978 1 85623 117 6

Disclaimer

The information in this book has been compiled for general guidance and is not intended to replace the advice
and treatments of qualified herbal practitioners or trained health professionals. Do not attempt to self-diagnose
or self-prescribe for serious long term problems. Heed the cautions given and if pregnant or already taking
prescribed medication, seek professional advice before using herbal remedies. In the event you use any of the
information in this book for yourself, which is your constitutional right, the author and the publisher assume
no responsibility for your actions.

So far as the author is aware the information is correct and up to date at the time of publishing.

CONTENTS

Foreword by Maddy Harland   vii

Preface   ix

PART 1   1

Chapter 1   Out On The Land   3

Chapter 2   The Wild Gardener   21

Chapter 3   Kitchen Medicine   35

Chapter 4   Seasonal Celebrations   55

PART 2   A SEASONAL GUIDE   69

Season 1   On the Edge of Winter   October into November   73

Season 2   Winter's Wild Edge   December into January   93

Season 3   On the Edge of Spring   January into February   111

Season 4   Spring's Wild Edge   March into April   127

Season 5   On the Edge of Summer   April into May   151

Season 6   Summer's Wild Edge   June into July   175

Season 7   On the Edge of Autumn   July into August   195

Season 8   Autumn's Wild Edge   September into October   219

              Cycles Within Cycles   247

Plant Reference Guide   249

Resources and Recommendations   281

Index   285

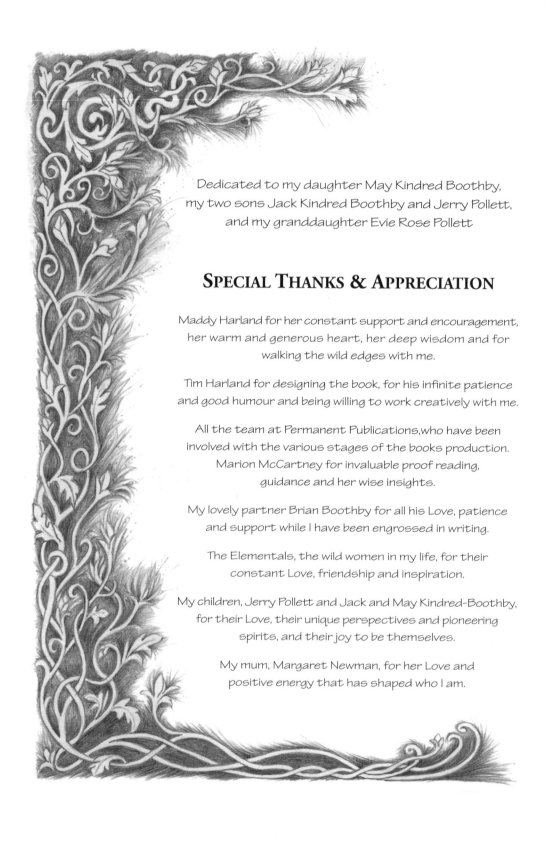

Dedicated to my daughter May Kindred Boothby,
my two sons Jack Kindred Boothby and Jerry Pollett,
and my granddaughter Evie Rose Pollett

SPECIAL THANKS & APPRECIATION

Maddy Harland for her constant support and encouragement,
her warm and generous heart, her deep wisdom and for
walking the wild edges with me.

Tim Harland for designing the book, for his infinite patience
and good humour and being willing to work creatively with me.

All the team at Permanent Publications,who have been
involved with the various stages of the books production.
Marion McCartney for invaluable proof reading,
guidance and her wise insights.

My lovely partner Brian Boothby for all his Love, patience
and support while I have been engrossed in writing.

The Elementals, the wild women in my life, for their
constant Love, friendship and inspiration.

My children, Jerry Pollett and Jack and May Kindred-Boothby,
for their Love, their unique perspectives and pioneering
spirits, and their joy to be themselves.

My mum, Margaret Newman, for her Love and
positive energy that has shaped who I am.

TESTIMONIALS

Letting in the Wild Edges touches on some of the most profound issues on the transformation of what it is to be human in a way that is unusually direct, engaging and deep... Our time in history is all about learning, as individuals, communities and a species, to respond appropriately to the crisis of climate change and the need to develop a culture and civilization, an economics and a politics, that is truly sustainable. At the heart of this is the birth of a newly oriented human being who knows in a mythic, poetic, philosophical and visceral way that Life is One. Letting in the Wild Edges contributes to this grand process.

Steve Nation, co-founder of Intuition in Service and co-convenor of the Spiritual Caucus at the United Nations in New York

Glennie's long green experience, wisdom and love for life emerge from every page, and the beautiful new pencil illustrations are more than an adornment: they add more layers to an already subtle and multi-levelled survey of eco-consciousness at the start of the new millennium. There are joyful things to do, things to gather and things to make – wonderful resources to harvest in your own personal walk on the wild side. Glennie has produced a bright, inspiring and green Book of Hours for our time!

Julie Bruton-Seal and **Matthew Seal**, authors of *Hedgerow Medicine* and *Kitchen Medicine*

Glennie's gift as a communicator of all things beautiful, celebratory, spiritual and practical is unsurpassed and this book is my favourite yet. Packed with precious and inspiring ideas to help us explore the edges of our worlds, it is must read for those of us who want to reconnect with the wild within.

Brigit Strawbridge is a campaigner, writer and speaker working to raise awareness of the importance of bees

The sheer joyful immersion in Nature's bounty which leaps from every page is wonderful to read. This is a beautiful book, a true compendium for anyone wishing to join Glennie in celebrating this unique planet of ours, in all its seasons. Superb!

Ark Redwood, Head Gardener at Chalice Well Gardens in Glastonbury, and the author of *The Art of Mindful Gardening*

Glennie has created a work of simple beauty, old wisdom and profound integrity. By encouraging us to expand into our wild edges she takes us on a journey that celebrates the full cycles of nature, gently pushing out the boundaries of what is familiar and leading us all, whether new traveller or experienced wayfarer, to examine both our physical and intuitive connections to soil and sacred landscape. While her detailed recipes and projects will keep hands busy, the effect of her book as a whole is to slow time, as we step into the ebb and flow of seasons and deepen our understanding of what it means to be custodians of the earth.

Carolyn Hillyer is an artist, musician and author from the wild hills of Dartmoor

Glennie Kindred remakes the connection between our hearts and our hands, our souls and the soil. With gentleness, wisdom and simplicity she reminds us where we come from and where our focus should be in these challenging times.

Sarah Pugh, permaculture teacher

From gardening to tincture making, from foraging to festivals, Glennie reminds us that the Earth patiently awaits our interaction and appreciation, offering healing on so many levels. Letting in the Wild Edges is glorious. A perfect and deeply nourishing sequel to Earth Wisdom.

Nicki an Greenheart, Wild Flower Essences

Glennie's deep love and resonance with Nature shines through every page in this book and ignites the wild self in us all. Informative and empowering, Letting in the Wild Edges gently encourages us to explore and experience the land as our ancestors have done since ancient times in a contemporary, co-creative form. It is an open invitation to take a wonder wander through its pages and to meet the wild soul of Nature for yourself.

Sophie Knock, Chalice Well Trustee and co creator (with Glennie) of the Plant Spirit Medicine Retreats

Letting in the Wild Edges helps us reflect on what is important and why. By looking within, by re-establishing our connection with the environment and by understanding its cycles, we might just find practical answers to global questions.

Saffia Farr is the editor of JUNO, a natural parenting magazine

Letting in the Wild Edges is a complete joy to read, and is so very beautifully illustrated. I urge you to take the hand that Glennie is reaching out – take it, open your heart, and immerse yourself in our wild countryside that has always been there, waiting for us. These are powerful edges indeed.

Jaine Rose, artist, writer, activist and recorder of life's wonders

FOREWORD

by Maddy Harland

So often we yearn for true connection with the land and its turning seasons. Our culture has taught us that we need to control and hold dominion over Nature and in doing so we have severed our intimate bond with her. No longer children of the soil, our lives demand that too much of our time is spent indoors. We have become conditional. We only want to be out in Nature at certain times of year when it is sunny and warm. We are afraid of her extremes.

Glennie sweeps all of this away. She urges us to fully, deeply allow ourselves to re-embrace the feral within ourselves. This is no intellectual premise but a journey in both the inner and outer worlds. She encourages us to get out on the land in all weathers and all seasons to forage, collect edible plants and medicinal herbs that ease acute conditions, to learn about our local landscapes, to meditate, or just be in the wild. We are encouraged to walk at the times of the 'edge'; at dawn and dusk, at the transition of the seasons, in groups, in silence, in wonder and alone.

Then she brings us home and teaches us how to grow a wild garden full of our native edibles and medicinals so that we do not have to rely on diminishing natural resources. Instead we invite the wild to our doorstep. We are taught to make tinctures, herbal honeys and elixirs, to craft from natural materials, to share food, and to anchor our appreciation for Nature in ceremony, both silent and personal, and with our friends, in groups. This is a joyful journey in the steps of our ancestors but with a strong sense of the contemporary. Glennie's seasonal practices, both pragmatic and energetic, lay a pathway towards a more permanent, lower impact culture.

One of my favourite aspects of permaculture is the appreciation of using and valuing the edge and the marginal. It has taught me that the edges of different ecosystems are the places of greatest fertility and biodiversity, such as the banks of rivers, woodland glades and estuaries. This is also where Nature's beauty is often at its height. There are also edges within our psyches. These are places where the imagination is most creative, where fear or joy arises unbidden, and times of transition between sleep and awakening when we are able to form impressions that dissolve in the full light of the day. These creative edges can also be found when we are absorbed in Nature, connected to seasonal cycles, transported by the intimacy of a special gathering or drawn deep by a symbolic aspect of ceremony.

As we explore the wild edges of our landscapes, the margins of the day, the shifting energies of the seasons in all weathers, and the turning of the year through its cycles, we heal a dissonance within ourselves. Too long have we yearned to truly reconnect with Nature, rather than being an observer. Here we learn how to let the wild edges in again and to open to our own ever-deepening connection. We are able to reach deep within our psyches and find our natural joy and power. We fall in love with the wild and the wildness in ourselves. Once we experience this wild love, we can no longer live in a disconnected way; re-acquainted with our heritage, we are freed from the spell of materialism for its own sake. This richness makes us want to preserve our beautiful natural world forever.

Letting in the Wild Edges is the story of this journey. It is a joyful, creative synthesis of both the spiritual and the practical, season by season. It is not only to be read and enjoyed for its artistry, or as a journal of activities and celebrations, we can live it too. This is Glennie's gift – her ability to navigate an ancient healing pathway – and to open a portal that we can all enter. In doing so we not only bring harmony to our inner lives, we reflect it in our outer actions. We deepen our ability to live more gentle, low impact and creative lives.

I have lived this book whilst it has been in the making and it has changed me. I invite you to walk through that portal and out into the wild edges and be changed too.

Maddy Harland
writer, editor and co-founder of Permaculture magazine
May 2013

PREFACE

In these changing times, we find ourselves living on the edge between the old and the new. We are moving into a new understanding that all life on Earth is functioning as one whole living ecosystem, and the Earth is an intelligent living being, a self-regulating, self-evolving, complex system. We can no longer perceive ourselves as separate from the rest of life on Earth, and with this realisation we move into the next stage of our evolution. This evolutionary shift into the holistic perspective is the great adaptation we are called to make for the sake of the Earth and for our own survival.

We have centuries of conditioning to undo and unravel in order to bring this new perspective into the reality of our everyday lives. The present ecological chaos is the legacy of the old mechanical worldview, which science no longer supports but which has influenced our society for hundreds of years and continues to be embedded in the way we relate to the Earth. This old conditioning has created our isolation from nature and our over-reliance on logical thinking, but this is now changing. Many of us are naturally bringing ourselves back into balance, becoming more willing to trust what our intuition, instincts and hearts tell us and returning full circle to the ancient understanding that 'what we do to the Earth, we do to ourselves'.

Society has changed too, becoming more eclectic and more open. We are mixing with people and influences from all over the world and the more we celebrate our similarities as people, appreciate our different cultures and learn from the legacy of the past, we move together as one people, to work together in harmony with the Earth, our unique and special home.

We are being pulled at a deep cellular level by the need to change but we are not always certain of the way forward. Change begins with joyfully embracing our willingness to be adaptable; trusting our instincts and holding out our hands to help others along the way. Change begins by opening our hearts and exploring under-used parts of ourselves, there on the fertile edges of our consciousness. When we let in the wild edges of our imaginations and our creativity, valuing the spontaneous and intuitive, we create a form of natural alchemy. This leads us to 'eureka' moments of illogical brilliance, as the spark of inspiration releases the creative fire of new solutions from which we can find new ways forward.

We, like the Earth, have a huge capacity to self heal, regenerate and grow. By encouraging our wild edges to flourish we engage our whole selves in the process of change and healing. When both sides of our selves, the logical and the intuitive are valued, we access deeper levels of our understanding. Where these two edges meet, our new holistic perspective grows. We learn through our experiences and from our experiences we change and evolve. It feels important to me that whatever we do, we must spend as much time as we can outside, engaging with nature, appreciating the wonder of the natural world around us. This will help us to stay grounded and keep us connected to the life force that sustains and nourishes us. Our shift into becoming aware of the infinite interconnectedness of all life begins when we make the decision to let down the barriers of our separation and experience the beautiful unity of life for ourselves. When we let go of our need to control nature and we celebrate nature's natural wisdom and unity, we move from being dictators to being co-creators. We are no longer separate but part of the whole.

This is a book about our relationship with the natural world, never far from us once we let it in. It encourages us to keep our feet firmly on the ground, to be 'earthed' through our daily relationship with the Earth beneath our feet and the web of life that surrounds us and is embedded within us. 'Letting in the Wild Edges' is about letting new things in, letting new parts of ourselves flourish and grow. To begin this new exciting adventure we have to let go of some of the old social and mental patterns that hold us back; our fear of change, fear of our intuition, fear of becoming too fey, fear of the dark, of walking in the countryside on our own and fear of using our wild native plants as food or medicine. It is time to let go of these old isolating beliefs. It is time to be open to the bigger picture and let in our trust. I encourage you to let your heart energy expand and create room in yourself for the wild edges of your intuition and instincts to flourish. These often neglected parts of ourselves are there on the margins of our greater selves, waiting for us to engage with them, to learn how to use them and bring ourselves back into balance.

This is a book about communication, relationships and inter-relationships. It is about our joyful expansion from isolation into the vast and infinite network of interaction and inclusion, as we expand into the interconnected web of life. Our present disconnection from nature is easy to put right. We simply have to want, with all our hearts, to find the pathways that reconnect us to the Earth, to learn to observe and to listen to the Earth and all that lives here as part of her vast ecosystems, and live with a greater awareness and sensitivity to this life force we are all part of. This is a call to be honest, true to our feelings, our hearts, our love, our growing understanding, and to be true to the joyful adaptation we are making. We may not always get it right and like any great journey it will have highs and lows, but if we don't set out we'll never know what possibilities there are waiting round the corner.

As we celebrate the Earth's wild freedom to evolve and grow within the infinite network of relationships and communication that is life itself, we recognise that we too are part of this same web of interconnected life. We are changed by this realisation and we can't go back to our old isolation. We become pioneers, great explorers of the web, dancers in the dark, expanding into the wild edges of infinite possibilities.

I celebrate nature as a wild untamed spirit, a tangled complexity of interconnection and diversity, a creative fertile force, interactive, intelligent, adaptive and alive. I have no desire to control nature, but to work with her. I see myself as part of the Earth, made of the same elements as her, and infused with the same life force.

I celebrate our pioneering spirit, our irrepressible ability to adapt and survive and put my trust in our open-hearted generous and caring selves, in our love for the Earth and each other.

I am filled with a deep need for a more honest dialogue with myself and the natural world… to expand, to stretch and reach out, to communicate with senses I know I have but have been ignoring.

I am expanding… no longer isolated but living within the whole.

I am expanding… and all my senses are alive to the subtle shifts in energy around me. I rejoice in my sure knowledge that I am part of this dynamic flow of life and connected to the whole evolving perfection and abundance of the natural world.

I am expanding… responding to my longing to let my wild edges flourish, to evolve and grow in ways that will help restore balance within me and in the Earth – for all things are connected.

Glennie Kindred
Spring 2013

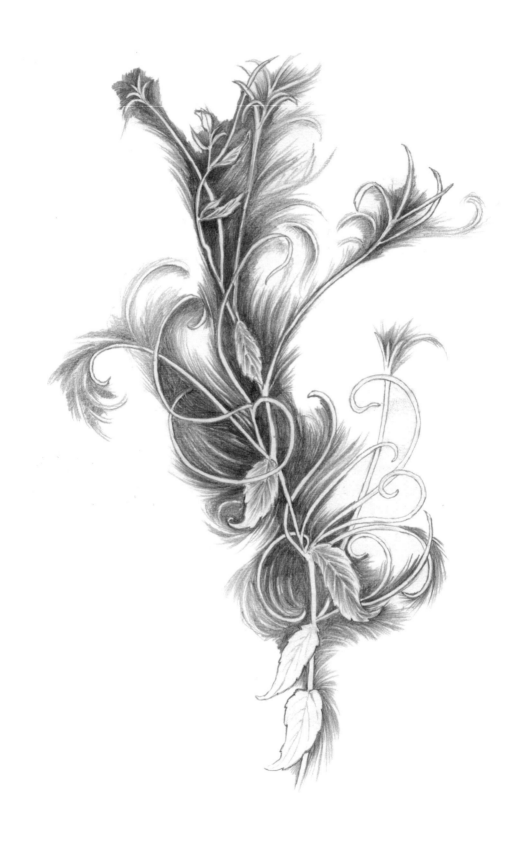

PART ONE

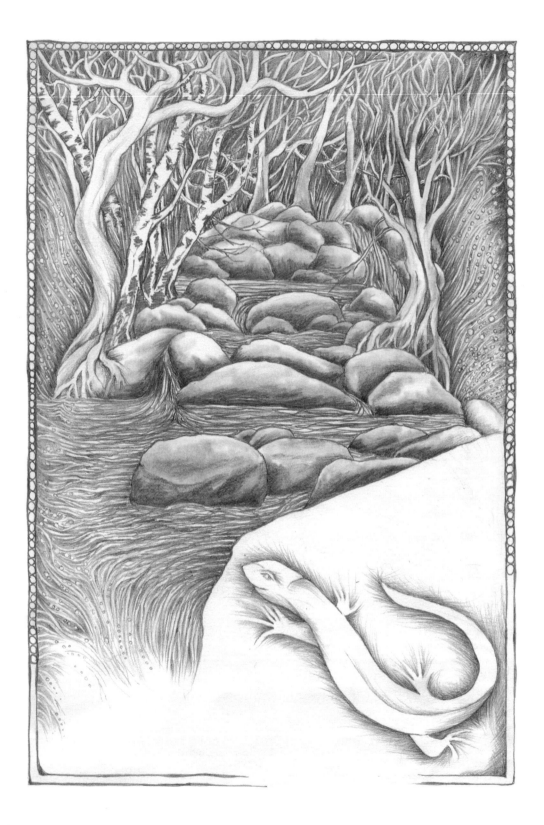

Chapter 1

OUT ON THE LAND

❋ Getting Outside With Nature ❋ A Tale of Separation ❋ A Tale of Integration ❋ Being Open to Adventure ❋ Extending the Wild Edges of Our Senses ❋ Valuing Our Intuition ❋ Restoring Equilibrium ❋ Mindfulness ❋ Time ❋ Sunrise and Sunset ❋ The Moon ❋ Electrical Earth ❋ Barefooting ❋ Pilgrimages, Vision Quests and Wonder Wanders ❋ The Native Trees ❋ Our Wild Native Plants ❋ Foraging

Like the Earth, we humans are diverse, intelligent, fertile, interactive and able to change and adapt in order to survive. As our Earth adapts to the climate changes brought about by our overuse of her finite resources, and the mentality that has brought this about, humankind is beginning a new evolutionary journey. The need for new lifestyle changes and changes in our thinking processes are tugging at us. The wild winds of change cannot be ignored and we must respond and above all celebrate this. We know that it is time to change, for the sake of the Earth and our continued survival here.

We are standing at the edge of a deepening awareness that everything here on Earth is interconnected and we all add to it, create it and are all part of this interactive, fluid energy flow. We are called upon to adapt and grow into this new awareness. In order to do this we have to courageously let go of the world we think we know and dare to be alive to the edge of the unknown.

Edges by their very nature are wild and fertile. They are in-between places, a mixture of the two systems that meet either side of them. They are places of dynamic change, the creative edge of nature's wild freedom and where this freedom is at its most fluid and adaptable.

By being willing to be open and trust the wild edges of ourselves, we make fertile a new kind of human being. By expanding our hearts and each of our senses, as well as our minds, we let go of the old view of ourselves as separate from the rest of life on Earth and become open to a new awareness of ourselves as interactive parts of the whole interconnected web of life.

Getting Outside with Nature

Out on the land is quite simply the best place to explore these new thoughts, feelings and sensations. Being out in nature is calming and reviving to our spirits, and the simple act of walking in the landscape slows us down and returns us to natural time. Walking helps our thoughts to flow and enables us to catch fleeting understandings as they rise to the surface from our deep natural wisdom. Walking is hugely beneficial for our metabolism as well as our wellbeing, helping us to stay grounded as we engage with the new and exciting frontiers of holistic thinking and experience a new relationship with the Earth.

So I invite you to begin this journey by deciding to frequently make time to be outside and to seek out the natural world that lives on the edge of where you live, whether you live in the town or the countryside, to seek out the wild edges where life is free to be fertile and self regulating. This doesn't have to be wilderness. Wild edges can be found everywhere once we begin to look. Once you have made your mind up to get out and find them, you will be rewarded and surprised by how much wild is still there on the edge of our lives. Along the railway tracks, along canals and rivers, along country lanes, roadsides (especially motorways), along hedge bottoms, on the edges of parks, in woods and copses, everywhere there are pockets of wasteland, forgotten and empty places, old industrial sites (check their history so there is no danger of any toxic waste in the soil), and overgrown gardens. We can also decide to garden differently and we let the wild edges thrive in our own gardens.

Decide to walk more often and find the routes from your home that connect you to nature's wild edges, places where you can sit with trees, reconnect to nature, explore your own perceived frontiers, push the boundaries of your perceptions and expand into the new holistic perspective.

Once you decide you want to make this journey, then the interactive life force responds, your desire and willingness to engage opens the door and the adventure begins...

A Tale of Separation

Nature lies all around us, at the edge of our lives, under and around all the concrete, brickwork and structures we have built over it. If we could no longer maintain our structures, or became extinct ourselves, very quickly nature and the elemental forces of sun, rain, wind, water and ice would reclaim them and within a relatively short time in the history of the earth, all that we have imposed on the surface of the Earth would disintegrate and eventually be reabsorbed. The wild native plants and trees are strong and resilient – they have millions of years' evolution behind them. Humans, on the other hand, are newly evolving and our journey here is just beginning.

Our desire to control the natural world began thousands of years ago, when we made the shift from being hunter-gatherers to being farmers. The nomadic tribes gathered their wild food from the forests, the lakes, rivers and riverbanks, the sea and seashore, the valleys and the mountains, and they respected the great diversity and productivity of the land and its life force. Each environment yielded different foods, medicines and other things useful to humans. Nothing was wasted, and everything was returned back to the earth to become reabsorbed and recreated. The people honoured the wild spirit of nature and gave thanks for it, for they knew themselves to be a part of its life force and the great web of life.

Our relationship to the wild changed when we began to clear the trees, and enclose the land to grow our own crops. At this point we became separated from nature. The wild went from being the 'great provider', to being something to be kept out, controlled and sometimes feared. The land became owned, parcelled up, divided, enclosed, given away by the power of the monarchy or the church.

The Agricultural Age saw the beginning of our disconnection, through the desire to control nature and make it work for us. The Industrial Age and Age of Science continues the trend, dominated now by the large petrochemical companies whose disconnection from nature is complete: deadly sprays that kill insects, birds, wildlife and the life in the soil; genetically engineered plants that do not produce their own seed and can contaminate other plants nearby to do the same; seeds that are coated with neurochemicals that indiscriminately kill all the insects that visit them, including the bees that we need to fertilise the crops. They are creating enormous damage to the ecosystems throughout the natural world. The need to impose control over nature has become so amplified, that we are now at this historic and unprecedented place of poisoning and destroying the very environment on which our lives depend.

A Tale of Integration

But now we are changing, standing on the edge of a new understanding. Information technology and photos of our precious Earth taken from space, have given us a broader overview. The science of quantum physics has verified the infinite interconnecting force that joins all of life together, which the tribes people understood so well. There is much to learn and much to re-learn as we begin a new journey of co-operation with nature and co-creation with the Earth.

Our new journey must begin with a change of mindset. Once we recognise our separation and our separation consciousness, once we see it and the devastation it has, and continues to, cause the Earth, we can do no other than turn ourselves around and decide to change. This is uncharted territory, and like the heroine or hero in the old folk stories we have to respond to the call to adventure, to gather together a few simple truths and set out on a great voyage of discovery. We take with us our great adaptability and ability to invent and create. By letting go of our old social conditioning of individual competition and financial greed, we lighten our load to freely choose, celebrate and value the gifts of generosity, appreciation, sharing, love and forgiveness as the means to change.

Being Open to Adventure

How many of us frequently drive past the woods or other places to walk, and tell ourselves we haven't got time to stop, even though we know we would benefit so much from it? Making time for our relationship with the Earth is also about making time for ourselves. We need to notice ourselves making the choices that cut us off from nature and we need to purposefully, with determination, make the choices that increase our opportunities to connect. We need to set our intention to be more spontaneous, to be willing to get outside more often and to be open to adventures!

Get yourself some good outdoor gear so you can enjoy being outside in all weathers – light waterproofs, good walking boots and a good well-fitting rucksack or day bag. A comfortable modern lightweight rucksack makes it easy to carry a few outdoor essentials you might need for a day out: a water container, salted peanuts, nuts and dried fruit, notebook and pen, sunglasses, hat, waterproofs, binoculars, scope or monocular, plastic and paper bags (for foraging), tissues, wet-wipes and a small torch. Keep the day-bag packed with these basics so that you can have an adventure at the drop of a hat!

You don't always need to plan epic trips – be open to what Roger Deakin called the 'undiscovered country of the nearby'. Find the wild edges of nature that are there, unnoticed right under your nose. Explore the idea that something moves between you and the natural world when you engage with it. Both are changed by the experience. Your appreciation of a plant or trees has a beneficial effect, both on the plant and on yourself. Through our open awareness of the natural world we become a little more alive to nature and nature becomes a little more alive to us.

There is so much to experience in this beautiful land of ours, so much to learn about and experience, so many wild edges waiting to be explored. Be open to the spirit of adventure, spontaneous days out, or jaunts to visit friends and see other parts of our rich and varied landscape. Ask everyone you know to show you their favourite and special places and invite them to come to yours.

Make a new intention to go outside every day, if you don't already, whatever the weather and no matter how busy you think you are. Go out in all seasons and experience the Earth in all of her rampant beauty. Become a weather-watcher and learn to sense the change in atmosphere and that coming rain brings, watch the clouds and be aware of which way the wind is blowing and what this might mean. Learn from nature.

Wild weather days are especially good to be outside in. Instead of hiding from the weather get out and explore the edges it creates. Change your mindset to seeing a wild weather day as being a gift, one to go out in and experience! Let go of your dislike of rain! It's beautiful! Celebrate it – for without it there is no life. It gives us our beautiful green land, our trees, springs, rivers and lakes.

Become a little feral, a little wild at the edges. Set out without destination, with a wildness in your open heart and see what pulls you and draws you along. Go out first thing in the morning, or last thing at night. You will be surprised at how good this makes you feel. Stand outside in the full moonlight, step barefoot into the garden, take your shoes off when out walking, find trees you like and sit with them, become a forager of edible wild food and make simple medicines from the native plants. Or simply step outside for the sheer joy of being outside – with the wind, rain or sun on your face, fresh air in your lungs, ready and open to see the beauty of life around you.

Learn to be open to the land, the forces that shaped it, its evolution and its past history. Places have their own stories, their own song, held in the stone, the lie of the land, in the plants and trees that live and grow there and which we can intuit and experience at the edge of our consciousness.

Stepping outside, going for a walk, connecting to nature, brings us back to Earth. When we are earthed and grounded we have a stable base from which to expand into our own wild edges and explore our new growing awareness that we are all part of the same interconnected and interactive life force. This fluid, dynamic, expansive energy-flow unites all life together and what ever we bring to the flow, through our thoughts, words and actions, has life. Whatever we give our attention to will grow. The more we expand into this awareness the deeper we experience it and know it to be true.

Learn how to be still, not just physically, but mentally and emotionally. Learn to listen to yourself, listen to the things you tell yourself and therefore make fertile. Learn to listen to your heart and your heart's longing. Become aware of your fears and the thoughts that inhibit your flow and expansion. Follow your joys and the thoughts that energise you. Breathe more slowly and deeply, slow down your metabolism and see what changes you can sense there at the edges of your perceptions.

Extending the Wild Edges of Our Senses

It is through each of our six senses that we become conscious of a relationship with the natural world around us. Our, eyes, ears, sense of smell, taste, touch and intuition are all natural parts of ourselves that we would have used much more fully in the past. Many of us have lost touch with them but they are easy to re-find and develop again.

When out walking, train your ears to listen more acutely to the sounds of nature. This requires inner stillness, melting into the background and becoming part of the landscape. Notice the difference in sounds as you step from one environment to another – as you step into the woods, or hear the approach of a river, stream or spring. Listen to the shift in sounds on the edge of coming night, or on the edge of a new day. Listen to the sounds that different trees make, the sound of their branches in the wind, the falling of leaves and fruit. Learn the calls and language of native birds and animals and have a go at imitating them. Recognise their calls to each other and observe what these may mean, learning their alarm calls as well as their songs.

Use all of your skin as an interface with each of the natural elements of Earth, Air, Water, and through the sun and light, which is Fire. Take your shoes off, take your clothes off, jump in water, mud, roll in the grass or down a hill!

Remember to engage with your sense of smell, and when out walking follow your nose when you 'pick up' a smell. Inhale the smells of the forest, the scents of trees and flowers, the smells of earth, the smell of the weather.

Learn the tastes of edible native plants, so that you have a deep and immediate contact and knowledge of them. Nibble them frequently until your palate welcomes their earthy flavours.

Use your eyes more fully, look closer and closer still, see how the natural patterns repeat themselves, read qualities of light, and learn to become comfortable in the half dark and darkness. Look far and further still to understand the inter relationships and patterns of the land and the landscape, its natural geology and history.

Expand your wild edges, dare to trust your instincts and your intuition. I urge you to be open to the possibility that we can establish relationships with trees, plants, birds, animals, and even a place. You may think that you are separate from that bird or this plant, but at a vibrational, energy level, a connection is made as soon as we notice them and especially when we love and appreciate them.

Celebrate the complete and utter beauty of it all, the wild abundance and fecundity, the great diversity and interconnectedness of all life at all levels. Our love and appreciation opens the energy for connection to happen, our indifference and separation cut us off.

Valuing Our Intuition

Most of us have not been encouraged to develop our intuitive sides and our minds are often so full of our own internal chatter that we are unaware of our intuitive responses when they do happen. They come and they go, and we often barely register them. When we do, we quickly forget them or ignore them in favour of the rational view. Our conditioned belief is that the intuition is not real, it is of no importance (therefore give it no time or energy), and it is not to be trusted or acted upon... When in fact the opposite is true.

Learning to receive and to trust these hidden and previously underestimated parts of ourselves requires that we look at our old beliefs about this, reframe them and tell ourselves a new story. Once we decide to engage with our receptive selves as well as our active selves, and learn to trust our own experiences and senses, the doors will open to this delightfully rich and natural part of who we also are.

Restoring Equilibrium

Listening to our own inner wisdom goes hand in hand with developing inner stillness. Meditation is a great tool for this and there are many ways to meditate. Basically, through meditation we bring ourselves to a point of one, and from there we are able to slip from the one thing into infinite unity. This one thing can be any thing – focusing on your breath, visualising or staring at a flower or stone, gazing at a candle flame, or repeating a mantra or affirmation. When thoughts do come into your mind, observe them (they are a window into your conscious and unconscious thoughts and feelings) and then simply return to the focus. Eventually you will find you have slipped out of time and entered into the stillness, the unity of all life and the vast internal web that connects everything together.

I like to do this out in nature. I find a spot that feels good... settle in... stare at something... slow down my breathing... and let myself zone out and become part of the environment for a while. This feeling of stillness I get from meditating out in nature restores my equilibrium and brings me to a place of inner peacefulness. I feel complete, whole, at one, and in balance. I continue on my way more fully present and connected, both to what is around me and to deeper levels of my awareness.

As these internal pathways become more frequently opened and used, the journey to this vital part of ourselves becomes more and more familiar. It becomes a known place on the edge of our consciousness, and one we can enter into whenever we choose to.

I find I can re-conjure up this feeling of unity and stillness wherever I am. I can re-call it, call it up – put myself back into the feeling. This is a useful technique for busy and stressful days. I literally remember what it feels like to be sitting in peaceful connectedness and breathe deeply into that feeling... and I am there! Just a few moments of this restores my equilibrium and connectedness. Have a go... It might take a bit of practice or you might find, like me, you can do it easily.

Mindfulness

Being in mindfulness is a Buddhist practice of keeping completely connected to the present moment, whilst going about your daily business. By being in the moment, in the 'Here and Now', we are able to become aware of our inner intelligence, grow with our hearts and become more receptive to our internal understanding. Being in mindfulness is an active state. It is not about sitting still and meditating but fostering an awareness of yourself in the present moment whatever you are doing.

Practise being in the present moment when you are out walking, when cooking, when gardening or harvesting plants. This brings us into a place of deeper connection and from here we are able to receive insights from the edges of our inner understanding.

Mindful awareness of ourselves in the moment allows us to observe the things we are telling ourselves, become aware of the chatter in our minds, and our everyday thoughts. The beliefs and attitudes we perpetuate in our minds are what we manifest in our lives, as all things are connected. Mindfulness helps us to see what we need to change in our thinking habits in order to move forward and grow in new and more balanced ways. We can change what we think, but first we need to see what thought patterns need to be changed.

Time

The introduction of clocks into our lives has created an efficient way for work hours to be counted and paid for in nicely packaged units. It keeps us synchronized worldwide, and is definitely a plus when catching public transport and keeping arrangements. It's convenient, but it is not the whole picture.

When we live outside of time and don't wear a watch, we quickly discover that time is amorphous, flexible and responds to what we are doing and where we are both physically and in our minds. Time speeds up when we are busy. Time stretches when we slow down and find our inner peace. We lose track of time when we are meditating, when we are creative, and when we become connected to our hearts.

Time takes on a different rhythm when we are out in nature and out walking. We expand into the wilder edges of our internal web, receive flashes of inspiration and intuition that can lead us to find creative solutions to problems and innovative ways to make changes in our lives. We are more receptive and aware of our intuitive selves, and are more likely to slip into daydreaming, which is hugely beneficial to us, shifting us from active mode into receptive mode.

Try having 'No-watch-days' and observe your change in rhythm, notice your anxieties, and your increased spontaneity and flexibility. Learn how to judge the time of day by the position of the sun and the light. Learn to let go of worrying what time it is!

Sunrise and Sunset

Understanding that everything in nature is cyclic immediately moves us out of the old linear way of looking at time, into an expansive holistic perception. We become aware of a vast matrix of interconnection, layers of ever-deepening levels of communication systems and the constant regeneration of the life force as it flows through the vast multi-layered unity of the web of life.

Much can be understood by observing the natural cycles of the sun and the moon. Sunrise and sunsets are special times to be out; even if you don't directly see the sun because of cloud cover, you feel and experience the shift in atmosphere, and often are rewarded by beautiful moments and reflected colours in the clouds. Twilight and dusk are edge places of heightened awareness that lets our instinctual selves come to the surface.

Get up before dawn and go early morning walking when most of humanity are still in their beds! Get a compass and find out where the directions are and observe how the position and time of the sunrise and sunset changes over the course of the year. Chart them from a fixed point by making regular simple drawings of the sun rising and setting in your local landscape, from your house or a place you regularly walk to, or take regular photos from a fixed point. The sun in fact only rises in the East and sets in the West at the time of the Spring and Autumn Equinoxes, when day and night are of equal length. At the Summer Solstice, the sun rises in the extreme North East and sets in the extreme North West. At the Winter Solstice it rises in the extreme South East and sets in the extreme South West. But it is no good me telling you this. You have to chart it, observe it and experience it for yourself to really know and understand it.

The Moon

The same with the moon cycle – you have to observe it and chart it from a fixed point to understand the moon's cycle fully for yourself. Become aware of the moon's monthly cycle from the dark moon to the full moon and its changing position and shape in the sky. Make a point of getting outside at night and looking for the moon or guessing where it might be on a cloudy night.

On nights when the moon is full, when you can see to walk about, feel your night senses come alive and the night sky opening you to the vastness of the universe we are part of. Light fires outside on the full moon, wrap up warm, eat round the fire, invite friends, play instruments, sing, tell stories. Feel yourself to be in timeless community, connecting to your distant ancestors under the night sky.

The moon and the night sky can be explored through a pair of good binoculars although there is much that can be seen with the naked eye. Learn about the constellations, and their changing position in the night sky. This was so important to our ancestors for navigation and a deeper understanding of the years cycle. Learn from the old myths and legends, and from astrologers. Expand your thinking to include a deeper intuitive understanding of the planets and their influence on our lives. Share what you know with each other.

Electrical Earth

The Earth is a huge battery that is continually being replenished and recharged by solar radiation from the sun, by lightning and by heat from its moulten core. We ourselves are a collection of electrical circuits; our heart, brain, nervous system, immune system, and muscles are all made up of trillions of cells all transmitting and receiving electricity. The heart is no longer being seen as an organ that just pumps blood around our bodies, but as an intelligent mind with neurological cells, a powerful receiver of the electromagnetic information that we, and all organisms on the Earth, are constantly interacting with. It is through our hearts that we communicate and interpret the world around us at these subtle levels.

All living things draw in energy from the Earth through their feet, paws and roots. The sole of the human foot has about 1,600 nerve endings per square inch, more than any where else on the body. We have walked on the Earth for millions of years with our feet drawing up the Earth's beneficial electrical energy in the form of free electrons. These equalise and reset our biological clock to the pulse of the Earth, which emanates a rhythmic pulse that keeps everything on the planet connected and in balance.

This contact with the Earth has been a constant for humankind for millions of years. We have walked, slept and lived close to the Earth, absorbing the beneficial electrical pulses through the soles of our feet, but in the last 150 years or so we have become disconnected from these beneficial energies by the introduction of rubber and plastic footwear, neither of which conduct electricity. The wooden floorboards in our houses also disconnect us, and on top of that we now sleep in beds raised off the ground, on the second floor or even higher.

Barefooting

Try to go outside every day and take your shoes off, especially in wet grass. If you are not used to barefoot walking, it will take a little time for your feet to become used to it and for you to gain confidence. Practise first at home and in the garden. Even half an hour a day is beneficial.

When out walking look for places where you can take off your shoes and walk easily in the grass. Include in your day bag a sturdy plastic bag to put your shoes in, some bio wet wipes and a small piece of cloth or towelling so that you can wipe your feet when you are ready to put your socks and shoes back on. This makes it easy to enjoy this sensuous and beneficial contact with the Earth and to make it part of your connection to the land. Find places where you can lie on the surface of the Earth for half an hour or more, making sure that your clothes and blanket are made of natural materials.

These simple connections to the Earth will help restore and maintain the body's natural electrical state. It is hugely reviving and restores us to a more primitive and instinctual edge. It is especially beneficial for the immune system and when there is inflammation and pain in the body. It will help with insomnia, anxiety, jetlag and whenever you feel tired or weakened by stress.

Pilgrimages, Vision Quests and Wonder Wanders

These are all trips out on the land with a special focus or intention. They can be done alone or with friends who are willing to hold and maintain the focus of the day, agree not to chatter and to walk in stillness and connection.

Pilgrimages are contemplative walks to a sacred spot, or a place that is special to you. They are usually done in silence and encourage spiritual expansion and reflection. You may be focused on a particular prayer, purpose or intention, and may include personal ritual, such as acknowledging and marking a completion, a new beginning or place of transition in your life.

Vision Quests are a contemplative walks, usually all day, usually alone, seeking an answer to a question of the heart. All kinds of signs and messages from nature and spirit are observed along the way, which add to the understanding and insights gained. Usually, only water, fruit and nuts are carried to eat and drink.

Wonder Wanders are a day's walk in nature, from dawn until dusk, keeping focused, as far as possible, on the here and now and walking in mindful awareness of the Earth, its beauty and perfection. A group of people can decide to have a Wonder Wander together but they must agree not to speak, unless it is to share wonder or to decide which way to go, or when to stop, eat and rest. Everyone carries their own water, food to share, a notebook to write or sketch in, and something to sit on. It is a day of aimless wandering, intuitive insights and impromptu decisions.

There is usually one person who facilitates, who at the bottom of their bag has a watch, a mobile phone, and carries a map, if possible only to be consulted at the end of the day. Everyone else leaves them behind for the day and so are free to fully engage with the natural world. The facilitator may also bring inspirational readings to focus connection to the Earth, and reads these along the way. Special moments are savoured such as the sun rise and the sun set.

The facilitator decides when to finish the Wonder Wander, gets the map out and at this point everyone can speak again and see where they have wandered and decide on the route back. It is especially good if someone can be contacted at this point to put on bake potatoes and a simple supper and if it is a fine evening, to have an outdoor fire ready for your return.

Wonder Wanders are hugely enjoyable and expansive adventures, creating deep connection to the Earth and the natural world. They have been developed by Marion McCartney and are inspired by her experience of Muir treks.

Inspiring Websites, page 284

The Native Trees

If we left the wild to re-establish itself unmanaged, the most noticeable thing would be the increase in trees, especially the native trees that have evolved here in these lands for millions of years, alongside the native plants and alongside humankind. For 400 million years trees have created the oxygen-rich environment that is essential to life on Earth as we know it today. They regulate the climate, moving water around the planet by drawing it up from beneath the ground and moving it into the atmosphere. They are huge converters of carbon dioxide creating the oxygen-rich air we need. Without them the Earth would not be the Earth as we know it and we as a species would not be here.

Being with trees is a very great pleasure I never tire of. Their beauty and ancient wisdom is immediate and accessible. They are great communicators. They influence us, if we let them. When we walk amongst trees our energy changes and we slow down. Our contact with the trees restores us to natural time and when we sit with our backs to them, we become more balanced and aligned to the natural rhythm of the Earth.

Being in the woods is so good for us, not only because we become more connected to nature, but because the woodland is filled with the oxygen rich air we receive from the trees. The trees are also bringing up nutrients and minerals from deep within the Earth and releasing them into the atmosphere through their leaves. When we breathe deeply amongst the trees, we take these beneficial trace elements into our bodies too.

Our Wild Native Plants

Our native plants have been used as food and medicine by humankind since the earliest times and were used extensively in this country until the industrial revolution took people from the countryside into the towns, and disconnected them from their roots. The birth of modern medicines, along with the ability to mass produce them has also added to this. But times change and there are many people now who are empowering themselves to understand their own bodies, and are aware of preventative medicine as the route to good health and natural wellbeing.

Many of our most common wild native plants are the tonic herbs, which boost the body's defences and immune systems. Many are adaptogens, which trigger the body to adapt and heal itself. In the past these would have been eaten extensively as native salad plants, added to stews and soups and eaten as wild greens. Reclaiming our love, respect and knowledge of these plants is an exciting and empowering journey. They have become greatly depleted in our countryside by the mass use of herbicides and by the mindset of those that perceive them as weeds, and not as food, medicine, and a valuable part of the whole ecosystem. But their seeds still survive and they can be found growing in places where nature is regenerating, such as old quarries, nature reserves, reservoirs, along the hedgerows and lanes and where ever they are left to flower. Many are on the endangered species red list, but many are making a comeback as our attitudes towards them are changing and we too add our influence to the whole.

Foraging

When we gather food and medicines from our locality we become more rooted in our local landscape. We become a little wild at the edges, and empowered by our reclaiming of what was once common knowledge. Once you start on this journey you will see native plants growing all around you everywhere – in friends' gardens, along the hedgerows, on the edge of the woods, along the edges of the lanes, on the edges of fields, along old canal banks and railway tracks, along the river banks, on wastelands – all the forgotten places, where native plants are free to grow.

Remember that all land is owned by someone and although most farmers will not mind a bit of hedgerow foraging, it is still worth considering this if you collect anything else. It is illegal to dig plants up without permission and illegal to pick wild flowers. Having said this, if you apply commonsense and don't over-pick or damage anything it should not be a problem. If you can find the owner and ask permission, this is undoubtedly the best policy.

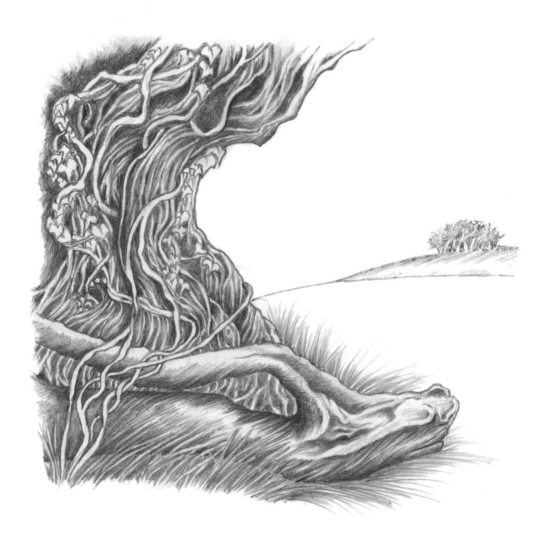

Foraging from farm land can also have other problems, because you must be sure that the land has not been sprayed with chemicals. It is also best to avoid industrial sites where the land may be contaminated. Here it is important to listen to your intuition and to only pick what you are one hundred percent sure of. The golden rule is: if there is the slightest doubt in your mind, then don't pick.

Map the native plants within walking distance of your home to see what you could use should you need it medicinally, or so that you can collect the seeds in the autumn should you decide to grow it into your garden or allotment. As part of your guerilla gardening activities decide to plant out more of the wild plants that you forage, thereby adding to the foraging opportunities for the future.

In Part Two of the book, each of the 'Out On The Land' sections has a seasonal focus for foraging and the 'Wild Gardener' sections have a seasonal guerrilla gardening section. We can also choose to let the native plants grow in our gardens, no longer calling them weeds, no longer wanting to eradicate them, but looking at them as a natural resource, learning to work with them, and valuing them for the food and medicine they bring us.

Foraging, pages 41, 77, 114, 130, 155, 180, 200, 223

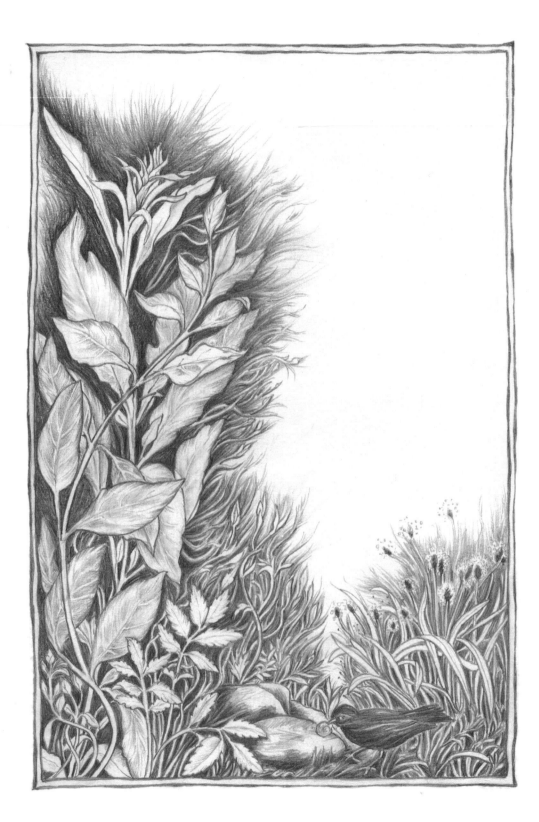

Chapter 2

THE WILD GARDENER

❀ My Small Sanctuary

❀ Our Changing Relationship With Plants

❀ Letting in the Wild Edges

❀ The Wild Gardener

❀ Growing Native Plants From Seed

❀ Shade Loving Native Plants

❀ Sun Loving Native Plants

❀ The Edible Plants

❀ Managing Your Wild Native Plants

❀ Insects, Birds and Bees

❀ If You Haven't Got a Garden

❀ Guerrilla Gardening

All of nature is essentially functioning as one intelligence, constantly creating balance in order to achieve equilibrium. The life force of our planet is inherently co-operative, and thrives on communication between all parts of the whole. The Earth and humans are a complex system. Once a simple change is introduced, a complex system will self organise, adapt, and bring all parts of the whole back into balance. We don't have to control it but only to understand that it will function as a whole unit, self regulating and constantly adapting to achieve equilibrium. With complex systems we can simply create the best conditions for growth, put key changes into motion and the system will do the rest for itself.

Our willingness to see all of life as a unified whole makes a difference to everything we do. We begin to recognise that we do nothing in isolation. Everything is connected and everything creates connection. We are inherently communicating and creating relationships through all of our senses all the time. This is how we grow, learn and develop. With this understanding we are beginning to realise that not only our actions, but also our thoughts and feelings ripple out into the interconnected matrix of life and affect everything in subtle and unseen ways.

The garden is a great place to explore these new understandings, to look at and challenge our old belief systems, to re-educate ourselves and develop our growing awareness of the interconnected web of life.

My Small Sanctuary

We all have different agendas when it comes to gardening, but the one thing all gardeners have in common is a love of being outside and a love of growing and nurturing plants. My passion is learning how to co-create with nature, to grow food within a self-regulating diverse ecosystem and to include the native plants as part of that system. I am aiming to create a balance between productive wild edges, thriving with native plants I can eat and also make my families medicines out of, and productive beds that keep us supplied with vegetables and fruit.

I have always loved the old cottage garden plants of our not too distant past and have always delighted in their ability to self-seed, send up runners, pop up in new locations and quickly fill a garden space with flowers without too much interference from me. The native flowers are much loved by the bees and other pollinating insects; they have after all, evolved together for millions of years.

Our native plants are incredibly hardy, many of them can be eaten and many are beneficial medicines we can learn how to use, yet we spend a lot of time weeding these wonderful plants out of our gardens! Once this realisation took hold, I find I can no longer go back to calling them weeds and I find myself planting the native plants that other people are weeding out!

The first thing I did in my own garden was to look at what native plants were already growing there and which ones I could eat or had medicinal properties. I began randomly adding the edibles in small amounts to my food. They were, after all, right there on my doorstep. I then began planting more of the edible native plants and now I can pick some kind of edible green salad for most of the year round, becoming a hunter-gatherer in my own small patch!

My knowledge of the medicinal uses of the native plants is growing through my direct experience of them. Their extensive herbal and healing properties never cease to amaze me and the more I use them the more I value their effectiveness and their teachings. As soon as I begin to use a herb my knowledge of its herbal use expands and my relationship with the plant changes and deepens; I am beginning to understand that we do nothing in isolation and our native plants and trees are supremely good at helping us explore this subtle sensitive edge of ourselves.

Within the safety and privacy of my garden I am exploring my growing understanding of nature's interconnected web and breaking down the barriers of an old separatist belief system I no longer believe in. Belief systems change as we evolve and develop. There have always been times in our history when a new understanding begins to take hold. This, I believe is one such time, and I am filled with the need to explore and find ways to help myself expand into this new holistic consciousness, first with my rational intelligence but increasingly with my receptive and intuitive intelligence. I extend my awareness into the wild fertile edges of my known reality and push a little further into new unexplored parts of myself. I am learning to trust my experiences, my intuition and my instincts.

My love and appreciation of the natural world opens my heart, so that in the giving I am also open to receive. I extend each of my senses a little further and become more conscious of the previously unnoticed subtle levels of communication and interactive relationships I am engaged in with the plants, trees, birds and insect life around me. Yes, my garden has become a sanctuary: a place of safety for all that lives within its four hedges, including me.

Our Changing Relationship With Plants

By seeing ourselves in relationship with the plants, we move into a new level of understanding and coincidently begin to have experiences which confirm that interaction between us does exist. Our native plants that have evolved alongside us for thousands of years are especially communicative and co-operative. Most are able to heal and help us both physically and metaphysically. There is more to this story than meets the eye and once we dissolve the self-imposed barriers of our isolation and welcome interconnection – interaction and intercommunication between all parts of the whole – the old story changes and a new story begins.

The maxim 'Whatever you give your attention to will grow' is evident in our relationships with plants. If we give them attention, they respond. I have found that a plant in my garden grows fine while I am ignoring it, but as soon as I decide I want it for medicine, or food, as soon as I decide I really like it and value it, it suddenly takes off and grows vigorously, popping up everywhere! It has responded to my attention and appreciation! This is an observed fact and has happened to me time and time again. This feeds my growing understanding there is so much more to our relationship with nature than our old isolated separation thinking pattern had us believe.

Something magical happens when we love and appreciate plants. It's the same as when we love and appreciate people: they begin to thrive. Wild as this may seem to some, there is only one way to find out and that is to test the understanding out for yourself. Watch the difference in yourself and the change in the plants that you give your love and attention to… It's a wild edge phenomenon!

Letting in the Wild Edges

Organic gardens are fast becoming sanctuaries for native plants, bees, butterflies, insects, birds and other wildlife, which over the last 50 years have been increasingly excluded from their native countryside by farming methods that have worked against nature. With this in mind it is even more important that we let the wild edges into our gardens and create the environments and habitats they need. Nature, left to her own devices, will self-organise and create a balanced ecosystem. This is true from the greater ecology of the whole planet, right down to our own small garden patch.

Decide to be brave enough to garden in a different way. Get beyond the old 'tidy garden' mindset. Let the wild edges flourish! By letting the wild back in to your garden, you let it back into your life. You begin to experience its rich diversity, rediscover the beauty and wonders of the natural world and experience nature's ability to create harmony and balance. It takes a good 3 years for a garden to become self-regulating but if you can resist the temptation to spray those aphids, their natural predators will eventually arrive in force to gobble up what is, after all, their food supply.

Become aware of creating a wildlife corridor, so that your garden becomes part of a bigger whole. Find areas of the garden that you can leave untouched, such as the corners and areas furthest from the house. Throw rough piles of garden and hedge cuttings here to compost. This creates nesting places for bees and other pollinators, butterflies and moths and their caterpillars, grubs and insects of all kinds, and are places that a hedgehog may find and hibernate in.

Make a pond for frogs and newts with plenty of stones and logs for them to hide under. They will do a good job of eating slugs. Create plenty of habitats for the birds who will tidy up and keep populations of insects and grubs in check as well as delighting you with their bright-eyed presence.

Let the wild plants in so that you are no longer working against them but are exploring their uses and celebrating their medicinal and culinary value.

The Wild Gardener

The wild gardener is a new breed of gardener, one who works with nature's natural inclinations to self-regulate and create balance, by letting in enough of the wild edges to let natural ecosystems evolve.

The wild gardener re-thinks what we should be doing in order to be a good gardener and redefines gardening with a holistic perspective in mind, aware of the bigger picture and the interconnective web of life.

The wild gardener encourages the wild edge to flourish in the garden, lets nature's rampant energy thrive and find its equilibrium. The wild gardener encourages a diversity of native creatures, insects and plants, and lets nature do what it does best, which is to create interconnection.

The wild gardener doesn't tidy up too much but in the autumn creates compost heaps in out of the way corners, so that the insects can find places to lay their eggs and hibernate for the winter, and leaves seed heads and long grass and fruit on the trees to feed hungry birds.

This is a whole new adventure that is full of delight and surprises but do remember to keep the edges of your garden tidy for your neighbours who may not appreciate your wild edges invading their space.

Growing Native Plants From Seed

Once, not so long ago, our countryside was filled with flowers; every hay meadow, every lane, roadside, and woodland. They have become so depleted that it is now illegal to pick wild flowers or dig up plants from the countryside. We can change this by growing them ourselves. I hold the vision of their seeds blowing out from our gardens and the native plants repopulating the land again. We can also do some guerrilla gardening and replant them out in any wild edge place we can find. Nature will do the rest.

Many of the native plants have a long flowering season and will help the pollinators and the bees. These are the country plants of the old cottage gardens, the wild flowers, the old fashioned plants grown before the current trend for exotics, hybrids and imports. I am always moved by their apparent frailness, and yet they are the survivors. They have adapted and evolved here for millennia and are filled with the life force of these lands.

Growing your own native plants from seed is the best way to learn about plants and plant identification. You get to know the plants in all seasons, from their earliest shoots, their flowers, their seed heads and what their roots look like. This builds an intimate knowledge of the plants from your own observations and experience.

Native Plant, Seeds and Bulbs Suppliers, page 283

Shade Loving Native Plants

Many native plants evolved in woodland and are happy to grow in the shade. I encourage these to grow along north edges where there is not so much light. To encourage the birds we took down our fences and planted a tangled mixed hedge of native fruit bearing trees, including elder, hawthorn, dogwood, rowan, bird cherry, crab apple and holly. This creates plenty of nesting places and food for the birds. It is a lot more work than a fence but ultimately more exciting and full of surprises and wildlife. It has to be cut back once the birds have finished nesting, otherwise very quickly this hedge would become a small wood, shrink in size and lack light for any but the hardiest of woodland plants. I once filled my garden with small rescued trees. They quickly grew and my once large sunny south-facing garden became a small dark wood. I learnt from this experience that there always has to be a balance between intervention and letting nature thrive… and that trees need plenty of space!

Under the hedges I plant all kinds of shade-lovers, like edible and medicinal woodland plants, and any of the useful native plants that will tolerate growing in shade. They won't do so well here if they are meadow plants for example, but being native they are tough and will adapt to survive. They are forever finding their way out and pop up in places more suited to them. They have a way of working with me too, just as much as I work with them!

Sun Loving Native Plants

These are the plants that would have grown in meadows and along wayside. They like to be out in the sunshine. Many are the cottage garden flowering plants many of us love. Some are annuals, most are perennials and a few are biennials. Once established they keep on going and will self-seed, increase the size of their clumps and send out suckers to reach new ground for themselves. They are hardy, resilient, loved by our bees and pollinators, and many have medicinal uses.

They will self-seed randomly or you can bend the seed heads near to the ground to encourage them to stay in the same patch of garden. Alternatively collect the seeds and re-sow them yourself. They also don't mind being dug up and transplanted so the young plants can be clumped back together in the spring. They have deliciously wild ways and move themselves about the garden, setting up partnerships with other plants, and generally have their own wisdom beyond what I might decide. I am totally in love with them!

The Edible Plants

The most immediate and direct way to take herbs into our bodies is to eat them fresh as a daily salad. The native spring tonic herbs arrive at the perfect moment without us having to do anything. They are there just when we most need them as we move out of our more sedentary winter ways. They are natural immune system boosters, and natural cleansers that help clear out our systems after the heavier foods of winter, and are packed with the natural vitamins and minerals we need to kick start our systems into action. Chickweed, cleavers, nettles and dandelion are abundant spring tonic herbs that can be cut and eaten like a salad crop before you finally weed them out to make way for conventional salad plants. There are many more that can be planted and once in your garden provide you with edible native greens all year round.

If you find some of the native leaf flavours too strong, bitter or earthy, then mixed them with the blander and more familiar tastes of conventional salads, or chop them finely and cover them with tasty dressings and homemade chutneys. After a while you find you get to love their tastes and your body craves them as it responds to their healing and life force.

Managing Your Wild Native Plants

Native plants will go wild and take over your garden if you let them, so they need to be managed, especially if you don't have a large garden and need room to grow conventional vegetables as well. Essentially I treat them like a crop, which can be managed like any other crop. Different methods work for different plants, in different parts of the garden and at different times of the year.

Method One
Preventing plants from flowering (and therefore seeding)
This is essential when you are eating the leaves of plants. Once a plant starts to flower, it will put all its energy into making flowers and hence its seeds, and the leaves begin to taste bitter.

Pick and eat the flowers and the buds and add them to your salad. They add colour and another layer of flavour, but they must be added at the last minute as they deteriorate quickly. They can also be made into oxymels (mixed with honey and vinegar), herbal vinegars, herbal oils and tinctures.

Kitchen Medicine, page 35

Method Two
Keeping them confined to their own patch
Encourage them to self-seed and re-establish themselves in the same patch. Once the seeds begin to ripen, bend the stems over or lay them close to the ground to assist this. Any plants that grow outside of this area are dug up and transplanted back in their patch, potted up to give away to friends or planted back out in the wild.

Method Three
Weeding as harvesting
Dig up any plants that are growing where you don't want them… in other words weed them out. This is different from conventional weeding though, because

where possible you make use of the plants for medicines and food, so weeding becomes harvesting. Nothing is wasted. Sort out the good edible leaves for a salad or put them straight in a pot to sweat and lightly cook like you would spinach. They can be preserved in vinegar or honey, made into syrups or other drinks. Alternatively if medicinal they can be dried for herb teas or made into tinctures. They can also be put in plastic bags in the fridge to use later and will stay fresh for a few days.

Kitchen Medicine, page 35

Insects, Birds and Bees

The wild gardener lets the natural world thrive and encourages it into the garden by providing the habitats it needs. Ponds are dug, hedges planted, logs and rough compost heaps are left for the insect world.

I am changing my attitude to insects and no longer see them as the bugs that might eat my crops, but as the bugs that might eat the bugs that eat my crops! Everything is part of the interconnected ecosystem and I am learning to let things be and recognise that a greater natural wisdom is at work. Without a doubt, slugs and snails are the most challenging as they have a tendency to eat the cultivated vegetables I am also trying to grow but it is interesting to note that they generally leave the native plants alone.

Providing habitat and food for birds ensures that you have plenty of them in your garden. Apart from their beauty and the delight they bring, they do a great job of eating slugs and snails and other grubs. This is all part of a natural self-regulating environment.

Birds bring the wild edge of the natural world into your life too, providing endless surprises and wonder. I spend many happy relaxed times watching the birds, often being rewarded by them coming very close, while keeping their bright alert eye on me. I have a sense of our developing relationship and of increased communication and trust growing between us. These are wild edge moments I value so much.

By growing more of our native plants we help the bees. Bees like our other native insects and pollinators have evolved for millions of years alongside the native plants of this land. With an astonishing 97% loss of wild plants in the UK countryside as I write this, bees can no longer do their foraging in the countryside. In fact the countryside is the worst place for them with all the pesticides and insecticides sprayed on the crops. Especially damaging to the bees are the neonicatinoids. These are seeds coated with neurotoxins. They are systemic, which means that as the plant grows the neurotoxins spread throughout the plant and affect the nervous systems of any visiting insects and kill them. The bees also take the infected pollen back to their hives and infect the whole hive.

We can all help the bees by planting the native plants they love in our gardens and reintroducing them into the countryside and along any wild edge we can find.

If You Haven't a Garden

If you haven't a garden, then start growing things in pots, outside your door, in window boxes, on balconies or roof tops. Containers need watering more frequently, but with good quality compost and organic feeds, their yields can be impressive. You can be wildly inventive and wacky in what you choose to fill with compost – old boots, wellies, old sinks, baskets, crates lined with old

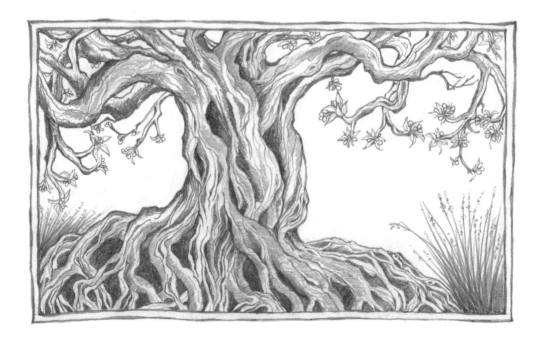

jumpers and cardboard to stop the soil falling out, old drawers, old buckets, washing up bowls, plastic bags held in place with logs, old bags and holdalls. Make drain holes in the bottom of everything you use because plants don't like their roots to be sitting in water.

If you haven't got a garden then see all of nature as your garden. Pay particular attention to the native plants growing in the wild edges nearby. Try using some of them for medicines and food. Engage with this rich heritage and resource that is growing all around us. Seek out all the edge places where the natural world continues to thrive. Help the wild native plants to thrive and become a guerrilla gardener.

Guerrilla Gardening

This is a movement that began in New York in the 1970s, when a group of activists and artists decided to 'green' their city. They took over abandoned pieces of land and grew flowers and vegetables. They encouraged anyone to get involved and together they created beautiful gardens in the middle of the city. The city authorities began to notice improvements in people's wellbeing and in the general look of the area as more people began to plant up planters and take a pride in their community. Eventually many of the guerrilla garden sites became permanent community gardens making the city a better place to live and work in. As a movement it has been spreading around the world ever since.

There are many different ways to guerrilla garden and many different reasons to want to do it. It may be that you simply love gardening; it may be that you have no garden of your own; you may want to get more involved in your local community and plant community vegetables and edible plants; you may want to improve the look of a neglected or run-down area; you may want to plant more trees or make more fruit trees available for all the community; you may want to help the bees and plant more of the native plants they love; or your passion may be to plant herbs and medicinal plants. You may work alone and unnoticed or be part of a larger more focused guerrilla gardening group.

My own guerrilla gardening passion is to reintroduce the native plants back into the countryside – for the sake of the native bees and insects, for the sake of the future generations and for those who are relearning to value their natural medicinal qualities, and for every walker and rambler who delights in seeing their return. Replanting the hedge bottoms, lanes and footpaths with

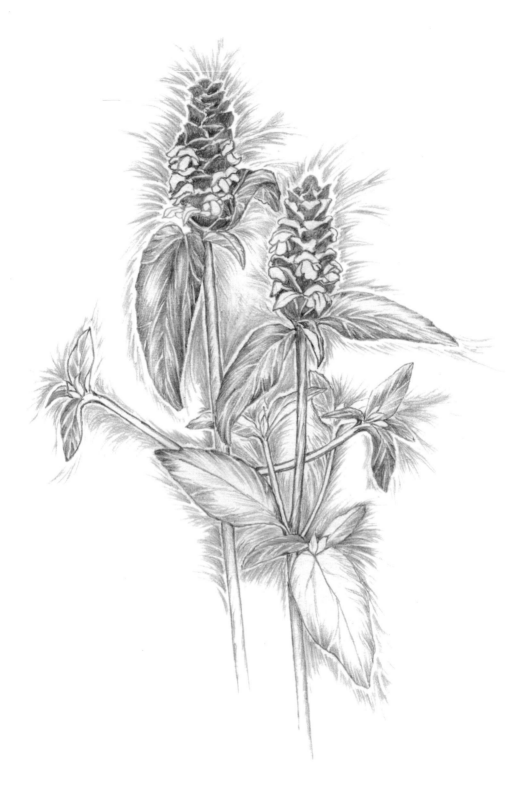

the wild flowers that once thrived there is my little bit of wild anarchy, my act of random kindness, my giving something back.

The guerrilla gardener is always on the lookout for neglected corners or grass verges, walkways, forgotten town planters, old neglected bits of wasteland or old car parks, small out of the way playgrounds, land beneath high-rise flats or abandoned pockets of land that are 'grey areas', with no-one particularly interested in them. There are always little corners that can be planted up with a few flowers or places that would benefit from a tree or two.

The important thing is not to become too attached to land that isn't your own, and to simply enjoy growing things there while you can. Just the simple act of improving the look of a place temporarily, and the enjoyment of getting your hands in the soil is enough. If your native plants have a whole season and go to seed, the chances are the seeds will find other bits of soil to land in and so their life will continue.

In Part Two of the book each of the Wild Gardener sections has a seasonal focus for guerrilla gardening.

A small Plant Reference Guide to some of my favourite native plants for the garden is to be found at the back of the book on page 249. It includes their edible and medicinal uses, their preferred natural habitats, gardening tips and recipe references.

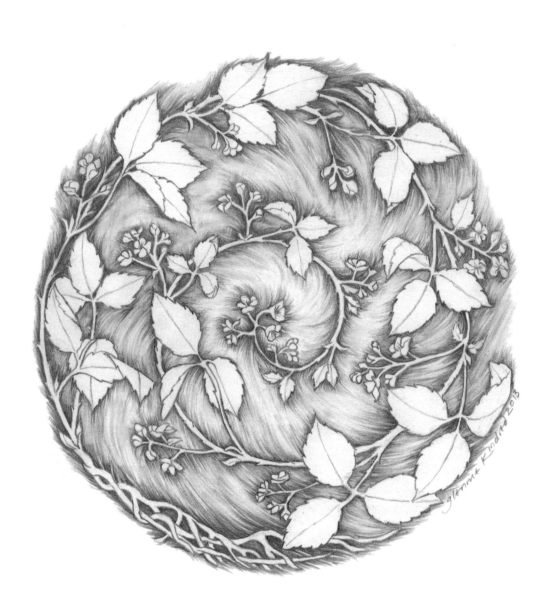

Chapter 3

KITCHEN MEDICINE

❀ Healing is a Holistic Perspective

❀ Making a Flower Essence ❀ Keeping a Herb Journal

❀ The UK Native Plants ❀ Harvesting Herbs

❀ Drying Herbs ❀ Storing Dried Herbs

❀ Making Herb Teas ❀ Dosage Guidelines

❀ Making Tinctures ❀ Making Elixirs

❀ Making Herbal Honeys

❀ Absorbing Herbs Through the Skin

❀ Making Herbal Oils (Macerations)

Using the native plants of this land for our own healing is to step into a relationship and partnership with nature. Our attitude, our appreciation and our willingness to engage with the life force of the plant all play a part in the healing process and help move us deeper into understanding the unity and interconnection of all life.

Growing our native plants and getting to know where they are growing in our locality, helps us to heal the separation between the land and ourselves. When we gather them and make simple medicines from them we become active in our own healing process. We also learn to love them, we take them into our hearts, and this creates a connection that heals our emotional malaise as well as our physical ailments.

Our reconnection to simple everyday medicine from the plants we have growing around us is empowering and beautiful and is a process of re-learning what was once common knowledge. They are part of our rich heritage and relationship with this land.

It used to be thought that the knowledge of these plants was gained by trial and error but studies of indigenous tribes today show that they use their intuitive faculties so much more than we do today and their knowledge of the plants is understood through a deeply intuitive relationship with them.

The medicinal uses of our native plants have been handed down for many generations by word of mouth and common agreement. Country people added the word 'wort' to their country names for the plant, marking them out as a healing plant. Later the medieval monks gave the plants Latin names, adding 'officinalis' or 'officinale' to denote that it was on the official list of healing herbs.

The great healer and philosopher Paracelsus wrote about their healing properties in the fourteenth century and his wisdom and understanding based on a healthy holistic perspective is still relevant today. In the sixteenth century herbalist and botanist John Gerard compiled his comprehensive herbal. In the seventeenth century Nicholas Culpeper's herbal included the underlying 'humours' or character of a patient as a method of understanding the type of plants to be prescribed. He also included astrology and the 'Doctrine of Signatures'. The 'Doctrine of Signatures' advocates that the appearance of the plant, the shape and colour of the flowers, leaves, seeds or root suggests its herbal use, a healing principle followed by country and tribes people and still used by herbalists today. Despite this illogical approach, modern research is validating the chemicals present within them and proving their effective ability as medicines.

In the 1920s, Edward Bach began to explore the metaphysical and subtle energies of plants and the understanding that the cause of illness lay in the emotional malaise of a person. He proposed that fear, anxiety and lack of equilibrium were the root cause of any illness, and that healing lay in restoring harmony and wholeness at the heart of the personality. His maxim was 'Treat the person, not the disease'. He worked with the plants at a deeply intuitive level and created a set of thirty-eight flower essences that are remarkable healers and still in use today, along with many more essences made in the same way and with the same ethos.

The legacy of these and many more great herbalists and healers lives on and understanding the different ways we can work with plants continues. In nature nothing is static. Many herbalists today recognise that the uses of a plant is not fixed in the past but continues to grow with our own evolution and needs. As we deepen our understanding of the interconnectedness of all of life, our relationships with the plants and the medicine we ask of them, are changing and evolving too. When we are willing to be open and value the healing abilities of our native plants, we can ask them for their help and work with them to create effective partnerships for healing.

Healing Is A Holistic Perspective

It is essential to look at any ill health from a holistic perspective, to look at the bigger picture and be aware of all the inter-related parts of our whole selves that might be leading to imbalance in the body. There are many things that affect our health such as not enough sleep; not enough play; too much stress; too much alcohol; not enough fresh raw salads and fruit; spending too much time indoors; emotional turmoil; not drinking enough water; dissatisfaction; despair; being ruled by fears; not enough exercise; not enough dancing; nor enough of all the things that makes our spirits soar and our souls sing!

We have to look at the whole picture. Like the Earth, our bodies are complex systems that responds to initial conditions. When considering our health we need to look at where we can reset the initial conditions by a change in lifestyle, behaviour, diet, attitude and beliefs, as well as our use of herbs. As the body adapts to the new life-affirming conditions, equilibrium and health are restored.

By living our lives with the understanding that we are part of a unified whole, we reset our initial conditions and enter into a profoundly healing journey with the Earth and all of life. As we become more aware of the interconnectedness of all life, we realise that we do nothing in isolation. 'Energy follows thought' in this interconnected holistic worldview.

When considering our healing, it is helpful to listen to ourselves, to the things we are thinking, the stories we tell ourselves, the things we say to others and the energy behind what we do. With this in mind, much of our healing is in our own hands. By changing the initial conditions and telling ourselves a new life-affirming story, we influence our thoughts, beliefs and attitudes and this creates a change in our health.

Remember to flow. Be open to change and regeneration. Let go of the old and all that drags you down and dampens your spirit. Move on. Don't get stuck. Celebrate your powers of regeneration. Our cells are constantly dying and renewing themselves, cell by cell by cell. The liver cells are fully renewed every 6 weeks, the kidneys every 4 weeks, the blood cells every 3 weeks.

Give thanks for your body and the power of the life force. Celebrate each and every day of this precious life. Choose to be happy. Healing is greatly facilitated by a lightness of being and a joyful generous heart. Laughter is a great restorer and nature a great reviver.

If you have a long term illness, physical weakness or debilitation, especially modern illnesses which are brought about by stress and stressful lifestyles, one of the best complementary cures is to spend time outside in nature. Take your shoes off and walk barefoot whenever you can. Appreciate and connect to all the beauty you can find around you. Beauty and connection to the Earth are powerful healers.

Making a Flower Essence

Essences are made outside in the sunshine, with the living emanations from plants and trees, which are at the peak of their power when they are flowering. They can also be made from a special place or a point in time.

Making flower essences helps us to meet the plants at a subtle level of their healing energy. They help us to change and heal at a deep emotional level and it is always a profound experience to make them. I have put this first because I know from my own experiences that our deep and subtle connection to the plant is essential to every thing else that follows.

Making essences takes us into our heart energy, helps us to connect to what is resonating from the plant, tree, place or time, and helps us expand into our intuitive wild edges. It is amazing what grows from these heightened moments, often bringing lasting awareness and understanding both of our own needs and the plant's essential energy and gift to us.

Method
You will need a small glass bowl, a small jug, a small glass bottle of spring water and a dark dropper bottle that is half-filled with brandy. This is easily

transported to wherever you want to make your essence by wrapping it all up in a cloth or clean tea towel.

1. When you keep noticing a plant or tree, and it seems to 'call you' to it, you know you need to make an essence. They are best made on a sunny day and sunny location. Admire the full beauty of the plant, and settle your energy with a meditation before you begin.

2. Fill a small bowl with spring water and place it next to the plant in the sunshine. You may like to put a little of the plant in the water but it is not essential. Sit close by but let the plant infuse the essence without your own energy getting in the way. Draw or write down any thoughts, words, poetry or intuitive understanding about the plant that comes to you.

3. You will have a sense when the essence is ready. This is purely intuitive but some times there is a slight change of colour, a golden glow, and the liquid seems to thicken slightly. Remove the bit of plant with another bit of the same plant and pour the infused water into a clean dark bottle half-filled with brandy. This is your Mother Essence. Save a little to water the plant with, and a little to sip with your thanks to the plant. Label the bottle and add the Mother Essence symbol (a circle with a diagonal line across it) and spend a little time decorating the label to spend time with the new essence and help anchor the plant's essential spirit.

4. Dilute 7 drops of the Mother Essence in another dark dropper bottle of half spring water and half brandy, and use (4 drops at a time) to help balance emotional trends in you that can lead to ill health.

5. Write up in your herb journal, with the place, date and insights you gained during the process of making the essence, as well as while you are taking it, noting emotional changes in particular.

6. Essences will keep indefinitely if kept out of the light.

Metaphysical Uses, Plant Reference Guide, page 249
Flower Essences, pages 38, 139,154, 179

Keeping a Herb Journal

This is a delight to do and becomes a very valuable reference book that is very much part of your journey with the plants. Choose a fairly robust notebook with a hard cover and plain paper. You can then make drawings of the plants, add photos or the pressed plants. Press them between pages of a large book (making notes of where!) and tape them in using wide clear tape. They can also be taped in directly using the fresh plant and a clear wide parcel tape. This works surprisingly well, but not if the plants are wet.

I usually have one herb per page. I write the date I picked it, where I picked it from and what I made with it. I add anything that I intuit about the plant as well as what other herbalists have to say about it. As I use the herb I add in my own observations of its medicine and my own relationship with its healing properties.

The UK Native Plants

This book is focused on the native plants of the UK, those that have uniquely evolved here for millions of years. Many of them grow in Europe too and a few can be found all over the world. They are suited to our climate, our soils and our insects, and have been eaten and used for medicine by generation upon generations of our ancestors since the first hunter gatherers walked these lands. I have used *Wild Flowers of Britain* by Roger Phillips as my guide as to whether a plant is considered to be native or not.

The other more familiar kitchen garden herbs, such as rosemary, thyme, sage, marjoram, fennel, garlic etc are Mediterranean in origin and are only briefly mentioned in this book, but if you grow them and use them in the kitchen, then find out about their extensive herbal properties and use them to boost the actions of the native plants. Bring the consciousness of their healing properties to your food and make medicines from them as well. They are aromatics so they can be added to remedies, teas and elixirs for flavour as well as for their herbal actions.

Some people have a deep fear of eating wild plants, and moving through this barrier is a great healing in itself, and brings a deeply profound reconnection to nature. If your fear is around picking the wrong plant, then start with the most familiar, such as nettle tops, chickweed, cleavers and dandelion. All have extensive herbal uses and can be made into an array of medicines.

Growing the native plants yourself from packet seeds helps with identification. Grow them as single species in containers and large pots at first, so that you get to know what the plant looks like intimately through all stages of its growth cycle. Remember to engage with the plants, talk to them and appreciate them. Pick and nibble them frequently so that you get to know their taste.

Choose to work with the plants you naturally like and feel drawn towards. Your love for the plant will open you up and create a natural affinity with their healing properties. Gradually, as you get to know them from the safety of your home, and you get positive results as you use them as medicines, your confidence in the plants will grow.

Harvesting Herbs

Before harvesting make time to sit with the plant, observe and absorb its presence and vitality. Check in with yourself how the plant makes you feel. Be spontaneous, let your inhibitions go and engage with the plant. Go wild! Have a conversation! Talk, hum or sing to the plants. This is what the aboriginal and tribal people do and perhaps you will find this easier than you think! It creates a joyful connection to our own wild spirit as well as to the plant. If you haven't time for a long connection, then simply take a moment before you pick them, to appreciate their vitality and beauty, and always thank them.

• Herbs are harvested when they are at the peak of their energetic potential. If you are harvesting the leaves, flowers, fruits or seeds then look for that optimum moment when they are at their best. With leaves it is just before the plant comes into flower; with flowers it is when they are fully open; with fruit it is when the fruit is ripe and sweet; with roots it is when the energy has dropped back down into them at the end of autumn. First year roots are the sweetest for eating; with seeds it is when they are fully formed and dried out.

• Always harvest on a dry day, when the sun or wind has dried the dew from the plants. This is best around midday or early afternoon.

• If possible take from many plants so that you don't deplete the whole plant's energy.

• When gathering out in the countryside, only pick where there is a great profusion of plants. Pick so that you would not know you had been there.

Leave plenty behind to flower and seed. Be careful that you know the land has not been sprayed. Cut sensitively with scissors or secateurs and place in brown paper bags or baskets. Never pick flowers from the countryside.

Foraging, page 17

• Bark should be gathered in very small amounts, and only if you really have no alternative. Be careful not to strip it all the way round the trunk or the tree will die.

• As always, write everything down in your herb journal: the date and where you picked it together with your thoughts about the plant and its uses. This is invaluable to look back on.

• Process the plants as quickly as you can. Strip the best leaves from the stalks and discard any leaves that have been eaten or have any mould, fungi, growths, eggs or insects living on them. Always check the backs of leaves for insect eggs or cocoons etc. Gently pull flowers from their stalks or calyx. Check over fruit to ensure you save only the freshest unblemished fruit. Everything else put back on the earth or in the compost with your thanks.

Using the fresh plant when it is full of its vital life force is best every time, but we have to find ways to store them so that they can be used all the year round. Drying leaves, flowers, fruit and roots is the most basic, natural and traditional way to store and preserve herbs.

Drying Herbs

There are various methods for drying herbs but they all require that the herb is dried and stored out of the light. I prefer to use brown paper bags, other people hang them up in bunches or lay them between sheets of newspaper or brown paper.

• If using brown paper bags always label the bags with the name of the herb, the date and where you picked it. This is good practice and a good habit to get into as plants can change a lot in the drying process. Even if you think you will know what it is, it is surprising how you can forget, especially if you bag up several herbs over a period of a few weeks.

• Leave the bags in a dry warm environment for several weeks. Put them in the airing cupboard if you have one, hang over the wood-burner or leave them on top of radiators. Shake the bags and turn the leaves over with your hands every day or two. It is essential to do this to stop any mould getting in to the herbs while they are still drying.

• The herbal properties of leaves and flowers will deteriorate after 1 year so they need to be re-collected every year. Fruit, seeds, berries, roots and bark will last for 2 years.

Storing Dried Herbs

It is light that destroys the herbal properties of herbs, so at its simplest herbs can be stored all year in brown paper bags, although if they are kept in the kitchen they will need to be kept in a plastic container or airtight tin to keep them dry.

Keeping the herbs in a dedicated leather or cotton bag is the traditional medicine way and these are hung somewhere warm and dry, near a radiator or fire.

Making Medicine Bags, page 192

Putting them into dark glass jars is good in a kitchen because of the condensation. Clear jam jars are fine if they are kept in a dark cupboard. At its simplest the jar can be kept in a brown paper bag or more creative ways can be found.

Making Dark Storage Jars, page 210

Making Herb Teas

Herb teas vary in taste and quality. Buying popular blends as tea bags is convenient, but be aware that the herbs may be old by the time you drink them, and the herbs may have been grown in monocultures and sprayed with petro-chemicals. It is infinitely better to make your own.

• Making herb teas is not an exact science, especially when using the common safe plants. Interestingly, different herbalists use different amounts. I use about a teaspoonful of dried herbs or a small pile that fits into the hollow of my palm, and between a half to a pint of water, depending on the need. Use less for young children and anyone who is weak and frail.

• Dried herbs have twice the strength of fresh herbs, so twice the amount of fresh herb is used.

• As you make the tea, say thank you to the plant. This open-hearted attitude adds to the healing process. I like to picture the plant and affirm its healing qualities as I wait for the tea to brew, partly to affirm the healing I am engaged in and also as a memory aid. This way I keep learning and understanding more about the plants all the time and keep my knowledge strong. Many of the herbs are an acquired taste. Nurture an openness to these wild flavours and earthy tastes and give them a chance. More often than not, a taste you didn't like at first becomes a taste that you find you love.

An Infusion or Tisane
Leaves, flowers and generally any soft aerial parts

Keep a special herb-tea pot for this. A glass cafetiere is brilliant for fresh herbs as the plunger holds down the leaves, and you get to see the beautiful colour of the tea. Pour boiling water over the herbs, and cover to keep in the essential oils. Leave to infuse for 5-10 minutes, or longer for a stronger brew.

The herbs can be left in the pot and topped up with more water and drunk throughout the day. Or strain off the herbs and keep in a glass bottle in the fridge to drink cold. Try drinking them from a wine glass or small tumbler, with ice or a slice of orange or lemon, or sweeten them with honey.

A 'Cold Infusion' can also be made with leaves and flowers by letting the herbs soak overnight in cold spring water.

A Decoction
Bark, roots, seeds and some tough leaves

Method One
Make a 'Cold Infusion' by soaking the bark, seeds or berries in spring water over night. Strain them off in the morning and drink.

Method Two
Crush or chop the roots, bark or seeds and place all ingredients in a saucepan of cold water. Bring to the boil, cover and simmer for 10-15 minutes. Pour the unstrained liquid into a jug and top up during the day with more hot or cold water, or strain and keep in the fridge.

A strained brew will keep in the fridge for three days. Discard as soon as it looks cloudy.

Dosage Guidelines

Dosage of herbs is something that those who are new to using herbs worry about. This is where your confidence grows with experience. Herbal doses are not always about exact amounts. You need to consider the type of herbs used, their herbal actions and the overall constitution of the person being treated. You need to be intuitive and keep a watchful eye on how the condition is responding to the herbs given. Always trust your instincts and take a commonsense approach. Large doses do not necessarily work better; in fact the reverse can be true. Modern medicine works with the assumption that we need instant results, but a slower healing process allows for greater understanding of the illness, and makes time for bringing in other lifestyle changes, changes in diet and attitude. All of this aids the healing work of the herbs.

ACUTE CONDITIONS
These come on suddenly and need more immediate attention.

Herbal Teas
In total 3-4 cups or wine glasses sipped through out the day.

Tinctures and Elixirs
A ½ to 1 teaspoon (15-30 drops) in water every hour or so, until the symptoms subside. (3-4 doses should suffice).

Herbs Absorbed Through the Skin
Herbal oils, or bathing the skin with the herbal infusion, decoction or diluted tincture, baths or footbaths can be repeated regularly.

CHRONIC CONDITIONS
These are long-term problems and are treated regularly over a period of time.

Herbal Teas
Drink 3-4 cups or wineglasses a day, for several weeks.

Tinctures and Elixirs
A ½ to 1 teaspoon (15-30 drops), three times a day for several weeks.

Herbs Absorbed Through the Skin
Herbal oils, bathing the skin with a herbal infusion, decoction or diluted tincture, baths or footbaths can be repeated regularly.

• Most minor conditions should improve within a few days and chronic conditions should show signs of improvement within a few weeks. As soon as there is improvement, gradually reduce the amount of herb until you feel the remedy is no longer needed. Switch to tonics and supportive herbs to restore the vitality of the body. Remember to feed the body with foods that will also support the condition and the healing process.

• For young children, the weak and anyone who is frail, halve the dosage.

• Don't give children tinctures and elixirs as they are made with alcohol.

• Generally it is not recommended to use a herb or combinations of herbs for more than 12 weeks at a time, because of the dangers of chemicals building up in the body.

• Obviously it is important to go and see a doctor, or registered medical herbalist if any conditions persist. Professional advice should be sought if the condition deteriorates and if there is no marked improvement after a few weeks.

Making Tinctures

Tinctures are the next most common way of preserving herbs. They are alcohol extracts that preserve herbs for many years. Tinctures work quickly as they are absorbed through the mouth's membranes and bypass the digestive system. They are also useful when we are out and about, at work, or when travelling.

The herbal properties of the plant, fruit or root are preserved in vodka or brandy or any spirit of choice. Vodka is the most usual spirit to use as it has no taste of its own but I urge you to buy one of quality as the cheaper ones may be made with GM grain or potato crops. I prefer the warmth of brandy, made from grapes or other fruit. The choice is yours.

The alcohol draws out the herbal constituents from the plant. A certain percentage of water needs to be mixed with the alcohol to draw out the water-soluble constituents from the plant as well. An 80% alcohol and 20% water ratio is usual for home tincture making. If using dried herbs you need more water but if using juicy berries then leave the water out. Home tincture making is not an exact science.

Method

1. Fill a dark jar with torn or chopped up leaves, sliced roots or crushed seeds. If you haven't a dark jar simply put a clear jar in a brown paper bag or clean black sock.

2. Top up with an 80% spirit and 20% water mix, and spend some time pressing the plant matter down with a chopstick or wooden spoon handle to remove any trapped air, which could oxidise and ruin the medicine. Put the lid on tightly and shake well. Label the jar and date it.

3. The next day, open up the jar and poke it again to release any further air bubbles. Turn the herbs over and generally say hello to your remedy. You will see that the colour is beginning to leach out of the plants.

4. Shake the jar every day or two in the first couple of weeks and thereafter when you remember. Open them up from time to time and see how they are doing, and give them a poke with a chopstick. Keep them where you will notice them but not in a bright light place.

5. After a month to 6 weeks, strain off the plant matter, being careful not to pour off the sediment that may have collected at the bottom of the jar. The plant matter can be strained initially through a sieve and then through a jelly bag, fine muslin, cotton, paper coffee or wine filters, which can be held in the sieve. Re-bottle the clear liquid into clean dark dropper bottles or any dark bottle, label and date them.

6. Pour a little boiling water over the spent mash, strain and enjoy your first taste, raising your glass to the plant with your thanks.

Tinctures will keep for 3-5 years in a cool dark place. But check them regularly and discard any that have gone cloudy or smell 'wrong'. If they have a slight sludge on the bottom they can be re-filtered using paper coffee or wine filters, held in a sieve, and then rebottled into clean dark bottles.

Generally it is best to make tinctures with one plant at a time and create combination tinctures later.

Tinctures are for adults only, because of the alcohol content. They can be taken neat but are usually taken in water, or fruit juice if you prefer.

Buying Dark Medicine Bottles, page 284
Dosage Guidelines, page 45

Making Elixirs

These are also for adults only as they are a mixture of brandy and honey. This makes them a most delicious way to take your medicine! They are especially good to use when travelling as they are kept in small dropper bottles and taken neat.

Elixirs are combination remedies, created for specific uses and personal needs. Elixirs need to taste good so the addition of any aromatic herbs improves the flavour, but must also support the over-all herbal action. They are experimental and fun, as well as being extremely effective and I like to give them creative names.

Write up everything in your Herb Journal. This is especially important when you make combination elixirs. Recording the plants and proportions used is invaluable when you create something you want to repeat.

Method One
1. Half fill a dark jar with a herb or combinations of herbs: tear the leaves, crush the seeds or fruit, and chop the roots. Send your thanks to the plants. Add a little of something that will give it a nice flavour such as rose petals, sweet violet, lavender, rosemary, lemon verbena etc, making sure that their actions support the overall use of the remedy.

2. Cover the plant matter with clear runny honey and send your silent thanks to the bees. Poke well with a chopstick to get out any trapped air bubbles and break the plant matter up further.

3. Then top the jar up with brandy and stir well with the chopstick until the honey has dissolved into the brandy.

4. Put on the lid and label, date and shake well. Give it a poke and a shake frequently and keep out of bright light. They are ready in about a month, although they come to no harm if they are left longer.

5. Strain off the plant matter and rebottle in clean dark dropper bottles. Pour a little boiling water over the mash of herbs that are left over, getting every last bit of goodness out of them. Toast the plant and its medicine and have your first taste before returning the spent mash to the earth with thanks.

Method Two
Create an instant elixir using the tinctures you have made.

1. Using a jug combine several tinctures that support the remedy you are making.

2. Mix in a similar amount of honey to tincture and mix the two together.

3. Pour into dark dropper bottles. Name and date and write up in your herb journal.

Their dosage is similar to tinctures, although I tend to use them little and often.

Buying dark medicine bottles, page 284
Dosage Guidelines, page 45

Combination Elixirs

Here are some suggestions of plants to choose from, depending on what you have available. I have listed the native plants first and the aromatics at the end.

ANTI-STRESS ELIXIR
Hawthorn, cowslip, vervain, rose petals, lavender, borage.

DROPS OF CALM
Hawthorn, elderflowers, cowslip, hops, valerian, vervain, rose petals, borage, lavender, chamomile.

BRAIN TONIC ELIXIR

For when you are working hard – betony, mint, rosemary, sage and ginkgo leaves if you know where there is a ginkgo tree.

PICK-ME-UP

Vervain, St Johns wort, betony, mint, rose petals, nettle, chickweed, rosemary.

DROPS OF LOVE

Hawthorn flowers, leaves and/or berries, rose petals, rosehips, chickweed, vervain.

SLEEP WELL ELIXIR

Valerian root, betony, hop flowers, elderflowers, hawthorn flowers, cowslips, red clover, lavender, thyme, chamomile.

DIGESTIVE TONIC

Peppermint, betony, chickweed, dandelion, hops, red clover, vervain, thyme, rosemary, lavender, lemon balm, fennel (especially the seeds).

IMMUNE SYSTEM BOOSTER

Cleavers, elderberries and elderflowers, nettles, self heal, rosehips.

FIGHTING OFF A COLD ELIXIR

Elder berries and elderflowers, self heal, yarrow, peppermint, chickweed, cleavers, cloves, star anise, cinnamon bark, garlic juice.

COUGH ELIXIR

Ribwort plantain, coltsfoot, chickweed, dandelion, elderflowers or berries, lady's smock, nettles, mullein, thyme, violets.

DETOX ELIXIR

Dandelion, chives, cleavers, nettles, vervain.

RESTORED ENERGY ELIXIR (IRON TONIC)

Nettles, chives, chickweed, lady's smock, self heal.

MENOPAUSAL PEACE ELIXIR

Lady's mantle, hops, vervain, rose petals, lavender, lemon balm.

Plant Reference Guide, page 249

Making Herbal Honeys

Honey draws out the goodness from plants so you can put herbs directly in honey and this makes it easy for children to take them. Not all native medicinal plants taste nice, so they can be flavoured with more palatable tastes such rose petals, lemon balm or mint. The herbal honeys can be taken by the spoonful, added to yogurt, ice cream or fruit, or made into delicious drinks. They are great to make with children, helping them become active in their own medicine making.

N.B. Do not give honey to babies under 12 months.

As always appreciate and thank the plants you use and send your thanks to the bees for making the honey.

Method One
1. The simplest method is to tear up leaves and/or flowers into a dark jar and pour on clear honey. Use a chopstick to help break up the plants and release their vital juices. Make sure there is no trapped air, which could cause oxidisation. Label and date the jar and write in your herb journal.

2. Leave the leaves in the honey and spoon out the plant matter and the honey to make a honey-herb drink when needed. Place a teaspoonful of the honey-soaked plant matter in a teapot or cup and pour on boiling water. Drink hot or cold.

3. Gently heat the jar by placing in a bowl of boiling water, strain off the herbs when the honey has become runny. Rebottle in a clean dark jar. Make decorative labels and date.

Method Two
1. Gather the flowers or leaves on a dry day.

2. Warm some clear honey in a bowl over a pan of boiling water, until it begins to get a little runnier but don't over-heat. Alternatively stand the jar in a bowl of hot water to warm the honey.

3. Lightly fill a dark jar with herbs of choice, tearing the leaves and grinding any seeds. Cover the herbs with the warmed honey. Prod well with a chopstick to remove air bubbles so that it does not oxidise.

4. Let it infuse for four to 6 weeks, stirring frequently.

5. Heat gently and sieve to remove the plant matter and rebottle in another clean dark jar. Some of the honey soaked herbs can be eaten, added to puddings or eaten on toast, or pour boiling water over them to make a delicious drink. Re-label, date and name your honey. If you are making it with children, encourage them to make a decorated label and give it a fun name.

This will keep for several years, although the honey will eventually crystallise.

Flower Honeys, page 188
Fruit Honeys, page 233

Absorbing Herbs Through the Skin

Herbs are easily absorbed through the skin. The fresh leaves can be placed directly on the skin or mashed into a poultice. The freshly picked or dried herb can be made into a herbal infusion or decoction and soaked in cotton, towelling or flannel to be laid on the skin.

HERBAL BATHS

Herbal baths are a wonderful way to relax and soak up the goodness of a herb and are an excellent way to administer herbs to babies and children. They are great too for relaxing tense muscles after work or aching muscles after a day's gardening. Make a pint of a strong herbal infusion or decoction and add to the bath water. (Halve the amount of herb for children and even less for babies.)

FOOT BATHS AND HAND SOAKS

Our feet and hands are rich with nerve endings that will absorb the herbs, again great for treating children who can always be relied upon to love any activity that involves playing in water! This is the same method as for herbal baths, but pour into a washing up bowl of hot water and soak the feet or hands for as long as you feel the need. Buy a bowl that is a good size so that your feet aren't restricted. Keep a bowl in the bathroom that is especially for this purpose. It acts as a reminder to have more foot baths! They are a total delight at the end of a busy day.

Infusions, page 44
Decoctions, page 44

Making Herbal Oils (Macerations)

When rubbed onto the skin, herbal oils will be absorbed into the bloodstream and the herb will act in its usual way. Dried leaves are best for making herbal oils. The fresh herb must be picked on a dry day to avoid mould developing. Only make a small amount at a time as the oil goes rancid after a while. Herbal oils can be made any time using dried herbs.

1. Place the plant matter in a clear jar and cover with organic sunflower oil. A cold pressed almond oil or grape-seed oil can be used if you want to make a massage oil that will be absorbed more easily into the skin.

2. Prod down well with a chopstick and place in a sunny window for 2 weeks, shaking or stirring with a chopstick everyday to avoid mould developing.

3. Strain though a piece of clean muslin and store in a dark bottle. Label and date.

If you don't have time for this or it is not sunny, then place in a double boiler over a very low heat until the herbal oil is warm and let the herbs steep for an hour or two.

Herbal oils are NOT the same as essential oils. Essential oils are distilled and much stronger and are generally not made at home.

There are many ways to preserve herbs, flowers and fruit in the kitchen. They can be made into herbal vinegars, cordials, infused spirits, wines, jams and chutneys. Recipes can be found in each of the Kitchen Medicine sections in the second part of the book. Each season brings new plants to work with as we engage with a deeper understanding of our own healing process and wellbeing and the gifts of the native plants.

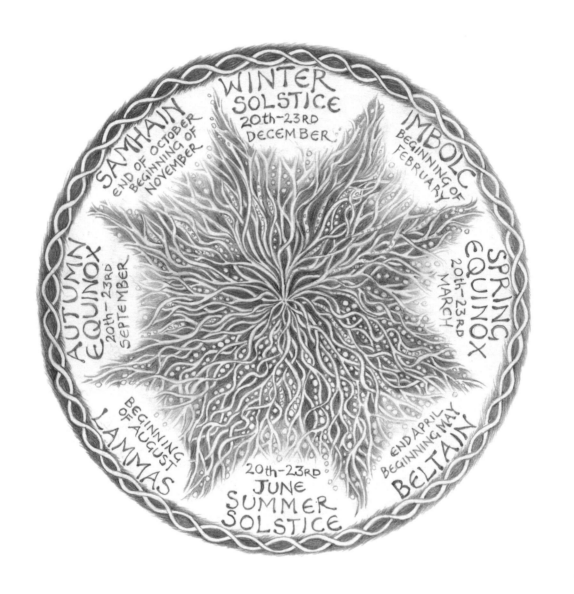

Chapter 4

SEASONAL CELEBRATIONS

❀ The Eight Earth Festivals

❀ Celebrating the Earth's Cycles

❀ Celebrating Outside

❀ Beginnings, Middles and Endings

❀ Celebrating Alone

❀ Co-creating Celebrations

The Earth has the ability to constantly regenerate and restore herself through her seasonal cycles of birth, growth, death and incubation. Each season brings gifts, opportunities and beauty into our lives in so many different ways. Celebrating and marking the seasons helps us to be part of the natural cycles and brings us into a deeper relationship with the Earth. By deepening our relationship with the Earth's cycles, we see that they are our cycles too. We are no longer isolated from her but engaged and connected. We become part of the web, integrated with the life force of the land and filled with a sense of our own belonging.

We have a rich heritage of Earth-traditions that have been handed down to us from our ancient Celtic past, coming from a time when humans lived much closer to the Earth than we do today. The 'Wheel of the Year' provided the people of this land with a yearly framework of eight festivals, within which the year's seasonal cycle was marked and celebrated. Although we would not necessarily celebrate them in the same way as they did then, we can use these ancient seasonal markers to deepen our relationship with the Earth, to rekindle a sense of reverence for life and reclaim our basic human need to get together in community.

The Eight Earth Festivals

The eight Earth festivals fall approximately every 6 weeks and help us to consciously align ourselves to the seasonal cycle and work with the prevailing energy that is influencing all of life, including our own.

Each festival gives us an opportunity to give thanks for the Earth and for all we appreciate and love in our lives. Each festival provides an opportunity to stop and step out of our busy lives, to step into wild-edge time, letting in our intuitive responses and catching the inspiration that rises from within us. They help us to become more in touch with our own personal journey as we look back on the last 6 weeks and see what is alive in us in this moment. From this review we are able to gather our new intentions for the next 6 weeks.

It is better to do something, around the right time, than let the moment pass you by uncelebrated. It need only be something simple such as having a special walk, visiting a favourite tree and sitting there a while to reflect and gather your thoughts. If indoors light candles, bring in some flowers or other seasonal delights, create a special meal, thank the Earth and the gifts of the season, write in your journal or simply gather with friends to share what is alive and strong in your heart at this time. Creating very simple heartfelt moments that can be appreciated by everyone is the key. Children love to join in with these and from simple beginnings family traditions will grow and friendships and understanding will deepen.

We can celebrate alone, with our family, with close friends in a closed group, or with friends and family in an open community group. (Or all of them!) There are no rules about how to celebrate, what to do or how to do it. Choose to do whatever works for you at any given time and aim to help all those present reach inwards to their own inner wisdom and reach outwards to each other.

Each celebration brings a deeper connection to the Earth as each person takes the time out from their busy lives to appreciate the gifts of the season. Celebrating with the Earth will change and evolve as your relationship with the Earth deepens, so start simply, with what you are comfortable and delighted by, and enjoy the way that your heart opens and your sense of interconnectedness expands you.

The Quarter Festivals

The Solstices and the Equinoxes are fixed by specific points in the Earth's yearly journey round the sun and are marked and celebrated by the four Quarter Festivals. These four fixed points in the year's cycle form an equilateral cross and mark the four seasonal heights of winter, spring, summer and autumn.

The Solstices

At the extreme edges of the sun's yearly cycle, the Solstices mark the shortest and longest days. Marked by our distant ancestors by stone circles, chambers and standing stones, they are significant points in the year's cycle that influences all of life on the Earth. Solstice means 'Standing of the Sun' and they are a moment of pause, a moment to stop and be aware of the 6 month cycle that has just completed and the 6 month cycle that is about to begin.

WINTER SOLSTICE
The Winter Solstice is the shortest day and longest night. The exact time and date varies slightly each year. In the Northern Hemisphere it falls between the 20th and the 23rd of December.

Winter Solstice, pages 103-109

SUMMER SOLSTICE
The Summer Solstice is the longest day and shortest night, and again the exact time and date varies each year. In the Northern Hemisphere it falls between the 20th and the 23rd of June.

Summer Solstice, pages 189-193

The Equinoxes

The Equinoxes are the middle points between these extremes of high summer and deepest winter. They are points of equilibrium in the sun's yearly cycle, when day and night are equal in length. Their exact dates vary slightly each year and they mark the seasonal height of spring and autumn. They act as a reminder to bring ourselves into balance, and to prepare for the seasonal extremes of the next part of the cycle.

THE SPRING EQUINOX

The Spring Equinox falls in the Northern Hemisphere between 20th and the 23rd of March.

Spring Equinox, pages 144-149

AUTUMN EQUINOX

The Autumn Equinox falls in the Northern Hemisphere between the 20th and the 23rd of September.

Autumn Equinox, pages 237-244

The Cross Quarter Festivals

Another set of Earth festivals are celebrated between the Equinoxes and the Solstices. These are the Cross Quarter Festivals. These are edge places, each marking a subtle shift in the Earth's energy as a new season begins to show itself. Alchemically, they are highly fertile times, power points in the year's cycle, when we can work with the prevailing power of the season and the wild edge of change and transition. They are the four great fire festivals of our ancient past, Samhain, Imbolc, Beltain and Lammas (or Lughnasadh), when community bonfires were lit on the high points and people would gather together from miles around.

Some people celebrate the Cross Quarter festivals on a calendar date. This is good for fixing the dates of community gatherings, and a fixed date creates a web of energy held by many. But for me, they are older than our Roman calendar and they are of the Earth, and have nothing to do with our human recording of time, so I like to celebrate them with a consciousness of the Earth's energy and the moon's cycle. A full moon gives a festival the thrust of completed power, strong emotional energy and moonlight for getting about. The dark of the moon or the new moon is more introspective and brings the power of rising energy and the potential of new beginnings.

I also celebrate them with an awareness of the Earth's own energy shift, and respond to when it 'feels' right. This purely instinctive feeling is a wild edge I value. I consider myself very lucky when I can spontaneously act on this, drop everything and have a wild-edge day outside on the land, absorbing the Earth's energy. I gift myself the time to reflect on what is alive in me right now and consider where I choose to put my energy in the coming cycle. Most importantly I feel myself as part of the Earth's cycle and connected to the whole wonderful web of life.

Samhain, end of October/beginning of November, pages 86-91
Beltain, end of April/beginning of May, pages 169-173
Imbolc, end of January/ beginning of February, pages 122-125
Lammas, end of July/beginning of August, pages 211-217

Celebrating the Earth's Cycles

By aligning our own lives with the Earth's yearly cycle we can consciously make best use of the prevailing energies that subtly and inevitably affect us all.

Taking a moment to celebrate or mark the seasons and the seasonal edges is different from just acknowledging them in passing. It means creating some focused time, shifting ourselves into a more receptive mode and actually marking the moment in some way. Celebrating the Earth, however simply, helps to anchor us in the here and now, takes us out of the mundane and lifts us into an awareness of the greater whole. It can be as simple as a dedicated day out on the land, writing in your journal or inviting friends to share in a seasonal celebration.

Each Earth festival is an opportunity to pause, to look at what we are feeling and what we can do to help the Earth regenerate and heal. Each festival is an opportunity to reaffirm new directions and let go of old negative emotional patterns that no longer help our progress. We can look at what we have achieved in the cycle just finished, both in the outer world and as part of our inner development, and set our intentions for the coming season. When we are more conscious of the new directions we wish to take, we are more likely to notice and act upon those unexpected opportunities that come from the universal web of infinite possibilities. Change comes rapidly when we trust the wild edges of life's benevolence.

There are many ways to celebrate the Earth's seasonal cycles. I offer a selection of ideas in the seasonal guides in Part Two of this book. These are things that I have found to work well, especially outdoors and in mixed community gatherings. They are inclusive and encourage communication, participation, going deep and having fun. They can also be adapted for celebrating alone.

There is comfort and security in repetition and you may find there are one or two things you like to do every time. It is better to start simply and repeat something that has worked before. It will come out differently each time anyway.

Beginnings, Middles and Endings

A little bit of structure provides the comfort of knowing what will happen next and a framework for spontaneity to unfold. This usually takes the form of a beginning, a middle and something to mark the end of the celebration.

• Creating a seasonal centre-piece, or central shrine is a lovely thing to do together before the celebration begins. Ask everyone to bring natural things to help create this or make it simply with what you find around you in the natural world. Traditionally each of the compass directions are represented by each of the elements of life.

• Earth is placed in the North: to give thanks for the Earth and all she gives us, the winter, midnight, going within, rest, nourishment, growth, fertility, manifestation, and is represented by seasonal flowers, seeds or fruit, stones, crystals, or a bowl of compost or soil.

• Air is placed in the East: we give thanks for each breath, the dawn of each new day, new beginnings, springtime, our voices, our minds, communication, and is represented by a chime, a singing bowl, a nest, or feathers.

• Fire is placed in the South: we give thanks for the spark of life, midday, summer, the sun, action, energy, inner fire, passion, spontaneity, trans-formation, and is represented by a candle or a burner for burning charcoal, herbs, twigs or incense.

Water is placed in the West: we give thanks for the water of life, the waters of the land and our bodies, the end of the day, autumn, the moon, flow, our emotions, intuition, receptivity, and is represented by a dish of water.

Spirit or the Web of Life is at the centre: we give thanks for the interconnected web of life, unity, Unconditional Love, our inter-dimensional reality, the spirits of place, our ancestors and descendants, our spirit guides, guardians and helpers, and is represented by a beautiful empty bowl, a vase of flowers or whatever feels right at the time.

Beginning a Celebration/Opening the Circle

How we begin a celebration sets the whole flavour. There are many simple ways to give people the chance to arrive and settle their energy.

• Sitting or standing in a circle means all are equal and everyone can see each other.

• Drumming and shaking percussion is a great way to mark the beginning. It is a signal for people to gather people together. It becomes a meditation and helps people to become grounded. A free-flow of sounds, tones and simple improvised tunes or phrases adds another layer of connection and unity.

• After this encourage a moment of silence, meditation, silent attunement or contemplation time. Other simple relaxation exercises can be added such as a guided visualization, grounding exercise (such as sending our roots down into the Earth) or an inspired reading.

• Light a candle at the centre with a blessing of thanks.

• Hold hands and have a quiet moment together. This creates a simple moment of connection, an awareness of the whole group and our collective humanity.

• Everyone takes part in creating connection to the season, to the place you are gathered in, and to each of the Five Elements of life. This is done through sharing words or sounds. When we make these connections honestly, bring them into our hearts, we see what is true for us, what is strong in us, what moves us at a heart level. By sharing our adoration for life we create a beautiful space filled with wonder for our beautiful Earth and our beautiful selves.

• Checking In – a talking stick or talking bowl can be passed round the circle. The person holding the talking stick or bowl is not interrupted. Invite people to say their name and what is alive in them in this moment. Each person brings themselves into the circle through this sharing and it gives everyone the space to feel they are part of the group and heard. When the person has finished talking, they say "I have spoken" and pass the talking stick or bowl to the next person. All agree to a Confidentiality Pact, so that what is said in the circle goes no further. Offer support and kindness where needed, but keep this very simple and brief within the check-in and follow it up later in the socialising time.

• As part of the check-in, people can say what they want to focus on during the celebration and offer any activities they have bought to share.

The Middle of a Celebration

The central activity can be decided beforehand, which gives people time to think about it and bring things for it, or a focus or idea can spontaneously evolve out of the check-in. Central activities are as rich and varied as our imaginations.

• Make something seasonal using natural materials, and trans-traditional craft techniques to create something unique to each person, filled with personal intention and focus.

• Seek inspiration from the natural world by engaging with plants, trees or the Spirit of Place in ways that encourage our intuitive and receptive responses.

• Make time to write and draw in your journal, to become aware of what is strong in your heart and mind, and to seek inspiration from within through meditation, writing poetry, inner journeying or guided visualisation, music, drumming or using oracle or wisdom cards.

• Encourage people to tell a story or read an inspired piece of writing or to bring an idea for an activity that helps creates connection and deepens understanding.

• Create a simple focused ceremony so that each person has the opportunity to leave behind the old and make new intentions for the present moment.

The End of a Celebration/Closing Circle

Agree beforehand on how you will finish and at what time and a timekeeper to ring a chime to mark the final stage. Endings need to be simple, heartfelt and expansive.

• All that is brought into the opening circle must be thanked and released from the circle. Their gifts are appreciated and the gifts and insights gained from the celebration are acknowledged.

- A song, a chant, a prayer, a dance, drumming or toning together create a sense of completion and helps everyone to connect back together.

- Pass round a talking bowl, talking stick, crystal or stone. This gives each person the opportunity to share the understanding and insights they have gained.

- Remind people to close down their energy centres and visualise a circle of protection around themselves before leaving.

- Drink water and eat at the end to ground yourself and bring your energy back down to earth.

Celebrating Outside

There is no better place to celebrate the Earth than being out on the land, so it is worth looking at how and where you could make this happen.

- The biggest hurdle to get over is the fear of other people who may interrupt you or judge you. Being out at dawn or dusk helps, as fewer people are about then. Celebrating with other people means there is a sense of safety in numbers. Another useful safety net is for one person to opt to be the watcher and communicator. This person stands on the outside of the gathering as protector and is willing to go and speak to anyone who might come by and explain to them what is happening. Alternatively the watcher will take part in the celebration but keep an eye open for any possible interruptions and be willing to break off from the celebrations to go and speak to people. Take it in turns to do this. I have always found that our willingness to talk to people is always met with respect and people seem genuinely very open to our celebrating the Earth.

- The weather is also another consideration and you have to be willing to be robust and accept the weather as part of the celebration.

- Within the celebration keep talking to a minimum – it is harder to hear outside.

- If you are out at night ask everyone to bring their own candle lantern and a torch. The torch is useful in the preparation stage and the lanterns create an instant circle to gather around.

• Fire is another great pleasure of outdoor celebrations. Arrange for one person to bring a lightweight Moroccan stove or any other vessel to make a moveable fire that is off the ground and won't scorch the grass. Ask everyone to bring some small pieces of dry wood with them. Wood can also be collected along the way if it is dry. Some places have fire pits already made, available for anyone to use.

• Celebrating at stone circles is accepted as people already associate these places with the Earth Festivals. Again it is good to have someone each time who is willing to talk to any members of the public who may be curious as to what is happening. The energy of the stone circles or other places of the ancients can sometimes be very intense. So be prepared for this wilder edge when celebrating there.

• Find a natural circle of trees in the woods within which to hold your gathering. To my mind there is nothing finer than celebrating beneath the trees! There may also be other natural features in the landscape that you can use as part of your ceremony such as caves, streams, springs or archways.

NATURAL THRESHOLDS, DOORWAYS AND ARCHWAYS

Each of the Earth Festivals creates a moment of transition, a pause between one cycle and the next. We can use natural features in the landscape to create a special moment and mark this transition, to step through as you make a wish, a promise or pledge to yourself or to the Earth. Look for things that create a natural threshold, such as a stream that crosses the path, or a tree down on its side that can be stepped over. Look for natural archways such as two significant trees standing together with room to walk between them or clefts in the rocks. Look for natural passageways where a row of rocks or trees makes a natural tunnel. Give these special places significant names as you build up your own mythology and stories around the landscape you walk in.

1. Pause and feel yourself to be part of the natural world around you and not separate from it. Take a moment to open your heart to love – for the natural world, for the Earth, and for yourself. Breathe deeply and settle yourself. Send your energy down to connect to the Earth beneath you and to ground yourself before you begin. Be aware of the interconnected web of life so that you know that what you are feeling, thinking and doing in this moment will ripple outwards and affect what happens next – as all things are connected.

2. Pause at the threshold, gather your new intentions, name them and step through holding your vision with certainty that it has begun.

Celebrating Alone

Each festival is an opportunity to take time out from our busy lives, to make sense of what has happened since the last festival and to decide what to take forward into the next cycle. If you can, take a whole day out for yourself, a retreat day, a day without a clock or a watch and with very little agenda, a day to practise staying in the moment and to let in your wild edges! This becomes a day that is different from all other days, a day to remember, one that unfolds and evolves in its own way, with whatever you bring to it, a day filled with unexplained mysteries, significant moments, chance encounters, filled with spontaneity, inspiration and a deeper understanding of yourself and the natural world around you.

It may be that you cannot make time for a whole day, or you only have an hour, or an evening. It may be that you need to stay quiet and at home. Whatever you do, make a little time for yourself and do what makes you feel happy and connected to the Earth.

• Mark the beginning with a meditation. Connect to each of the elements of life and bring them into your heart by giving thanks for the gifts they bring you.

• At its simplest, look back on the last 6 weeks, to what has touched your heart, the good things as well as the difficult. Bring your awareness to where this has bought you to in the present moment, and make new intentions to help yourself move forwards in the direction you wish to take. Use positive affirmations and intention statements to anchor your new direction. All of this can be written down in your journal as a dialogue with yourself.

• If you cannot get out on the land, then step outside anyway and see what you see and what you feel. Breathe deeply, smell the air, absorb the weather, find a tree to stand or sit with, take your shoes off, find simple communion with the natural world in whatever way you can. Look upwards and connect to the clouds, the sun, the moon and the vast cosmos above us. Send your love out into the great unknown. Send your love to those you love and count your blessings.

• Indoors you can light candles, give thanks for the Earth and each element that gives you life.

• Tune into the season. See yourself as part of its energy and flow. This will help you to explore the nature of new directions and the opportunities that each season has to offer.

• Decide to make something that represents your new way forward. Write messages to yourself on pieces of silver birch bark or card, decorate them and hang them in your window as reminders of your insights. When you have absorbed the message, take them out and hang them in a tree.

• Formally mark the end in whatever way feels right to you, thanking the elements and any connections you made.

• Drink water throughout and eat something at the end to ground yourself and bring your energy back down to earth.

Beginnings, Middles and Endings, page 60

Co-creating Celebrations

Co-creating celebrations help us to find our way into a new group dynamic, one that changes and flows each time, according to who has the energy and inspiration in that moment. They encourage equality. They encourage everyone to feel that they can speak their own truth and each person's truth is accepted as part of the whole. This means that a gathering can include people of all faiths and all faiths are welcome and included. In this way we become less judgmental, more tolerant and more inclusive. People feel held in each other's loving kindness so they can speak from the heart. This creates an atmosphere of joy, freedom and safety.

• The structure, form and content of a celebration are completely up to you. There are no rules, no hierarchy of anyone telling you what to do, or presets for what must be done! We are completely free to create the celebrations we wish to. Within the wild edge of infinite possibilities, it is good to have a few simple structures that help the ceremony flow well.

• Gather in a circle and aim to create a beginning, middle and end to your celebration. This brings a familiar flow and known structure that people feel comfortable with. Each person is encouraged to try out new ideas and to hold the space for others at different times.

Beginnings, Middles and Endings, page 60

• There are different considerations according to the season and the location, whether you are celebrating within a closed group of friends, or if it is an open community gathering that may include children.

• In open community gatherings have one or two people each time who are willing to meet and greet and make sure everyone looks comfortable and is included.

• There needs to be a prearranged signal so that the transition from talking and socialising to beginning the celebration is a smooth one. Group drumming and percussion, or a simple chant will bring the group together. It creates a meditative, connecting and absorbing beginning, so try not to set the pace too fast.

• It is good to have someone willing to be the timekeeper, to keep an overview, to be aware of the flow of time, to be willing to sensitively step in and move things along if need be and to make sure the celebration ends at the agreed time.

There are many different ways to celebrate the Earth festivals and many different ways to link in with the season. Any activity is valid, from walking the land to making a special cake; from spending time in the garden, making a remedy, essence or elixir, planting dedicated seeds or bulbs with intention, or taking a short walk to sit with a special tree. The important thing is to choose a moment, be it spontaneous or planned, with others or alone, and to be alive to that moment. Practise the art of looking inwards and outwards at the same time. Allow your wild edges to flourish and be open to your intuitive and instinctive nature. Put aside quality time to spend with the Earth. Remember to stop, slow down and appreciate all her infinite beauty and perfection, and your relationship with her will never be the same again!

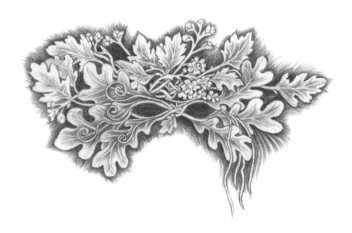

PART TWO

A SEASONAL GUIDE

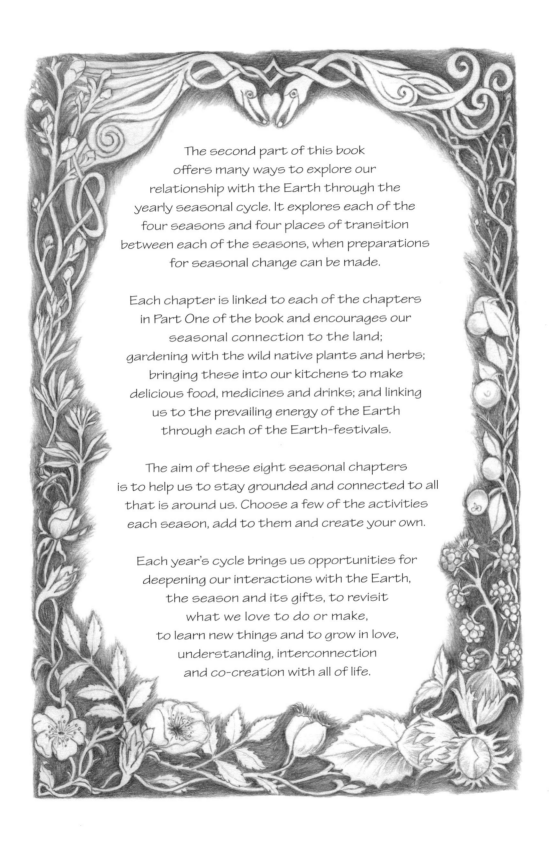

The second part of this book
offers many ways to explore our
relationship with the Earth through the
yearly seasonal cycle. It explores each of the
four seasons and four places of transition
between each of the seasons, when preparations
for seasonal change can be made.

Each chapter is linked to each of the chapters
in Part One of the book and encourages our
seasonal connection to the land;
gardening with the wild native plants and herbs;
bringing these into our kitchens to make
delicious food, medicines and drinks; and linking
us to the prevailing energy of the Earth
through each of the Earth-festivals.

The aim of these eight seasonal chapters
is to help us to stay grounded and connected to all
that is around us. Choose a few of the activities
each season, add to them and create your own.

Each year's cycle brings us opportunities for
deepening our interactions with the Earth,
the season and its gifts, to revisit
what we love to do or make,
to learn new things and to grow in love,
understanding, interconnection
and co-creation with all of life.

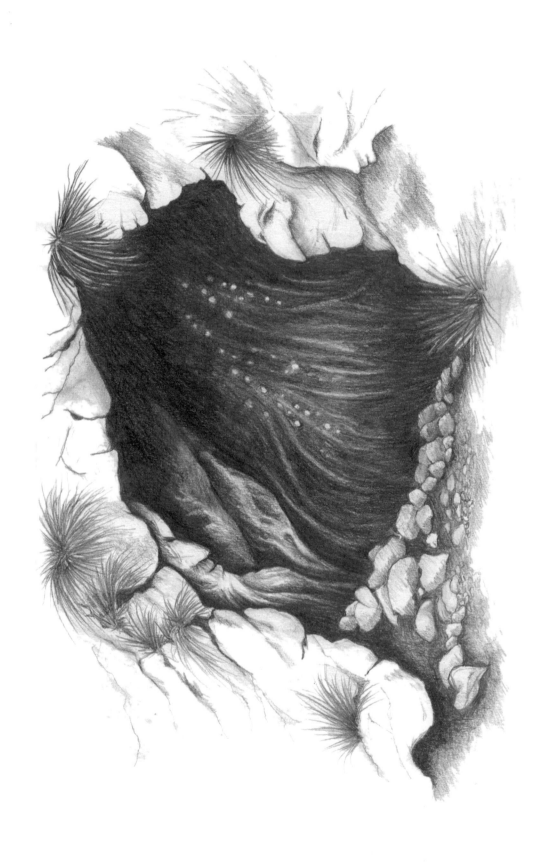

on the edge of WINTER

October into November

All of life is in the process of withdrawing now, to regenerate and renew itself by resting in the dark of the year. The plants begin to die back, and seeds dry and fall. The last of the fruit and the leaves from the trees are blown off in the autumn winds, everything returning to the Earth, to break down, decay and give their nutrients and goodness back into the soil.

Below the ground, the time of root energy begins. Roots have the power to break up rock and concrete and to make soil. They grow deep, seeking the minerals and nutrients they need to grow strong. Seeds that have fallen and are covered by leaves, waiting for times to change and light to return.

The weather is very changeable now, the days shorten and the sun is low in the sky. In between the many beautiful sunny autumn days filled with the bright colours of the turning leaves, there are dark, wet, cold days, when the mists come down and we follow our own need to withdraw, rest and reflect.

OUT ON THE LAND

✤ A Walk Every Day

✤ Day Bag, Walking Stick and Weatherproofs at the Ready

✤ Places of the Ancients ✤ Caves

✤ Commemorative Tree Planting

✤ Foraging – Gathering Sloes

The leaves gradually fall from the trees and each tree becomes surrounded by a sea of its own bright colourful leaves. As the trees are laid bare, the landscape reveals itself and this is a great opportunity to get a clearer idea of the topography of the landscape. Learn to identify the shapes that the different tree species make in winter, each unique and distinctive, aided by the leaves that are still on the ground beneath them. Bright green mosses shine out vividly amongst the increasingly brown landscape of the woods. The lichen are revealed, looking otherworldly and ancient, covering rocks and trees with their seaweed-like patterns.

We now have a real sense of being on the edge of the winter cycle. The Earth festival of Samhain recognises this as the ending of one cycle and the beginning of a new cycle. Like the Earth, it is time to rest now and nurture our seeds through the winter so that new life can grow from our deep inner longings. It is time to let go of the old year and dream new dreams in the dark. All life begins inside, in the dark, in the womb, in the ground, in our imaginations, in our hearts and in our deep intuitive knowing. Take this understanding with you as you walk the land.

A Walk Every Day

A walk every day becomes my aim, to counteract the tendency to be too sedentary at this time of year. If the sun comes out, even for a bit, then I am outside and making the most of it. It is a great treat to be out walking the land on wild weather days, to experience the wild richness and beauty of our ever-changing landscape. The early morning mists are worth getting up and outside for. Layers of trees and hills appear and disappear and if you are lucky, an intense golden sun can break through, causing the mists to lift and reveal what has been hidden. On clear sky mornings find places where you can watch the sun rise and stand in its glorious golden rays.

Day Bag, Walking Stick and Weatherproofs at the Ready

If you have a good waterproof jacket and leggings, good boots that keep your feet dry, and a hat to keep your head warm, then you can enjoy the wild weather this time of year brings. When out walking, be aware of the shorter daylight hours and keep a torch with fresh batteries in your day bag, in case you find yourself walking home in the dusk and the dark.

The landscape also changes as the rains return with streams and rivers swelling, crossing places are lost, boggy places reappear, forcing you to change your route and take a different path.

The weather can also change suddenly, fog can come down quickly, so keep a weather-eye open and let someone know where you are going if you go out alone onto the moors or into the hills.

A good walking stick is helpful in the winter when slopes can be slippery.

Making Your Own Walking Stick, page 215

Places of the Ancients

This is traditionally the time to honour the ancestors, so make a pilgrimage to an ancient site or burial ground. Put aside some time for reflection and meditation here, and see what comes to you. Ask for help from the ancestors as you make a commitment to help the Earth.

The megalithic monuments of the past were often marked by huge stones, which the people who built them sometimes felt compelled to move hundreds of miles across the land from one site to another. They may have experienced the rocks and the geological anomalies at the points where they were placed in a different way than we do today. Neolithic and Bronze Age burial mounds, barrows, tumuli, dolmen and fogous, often mark the sites of great geological fault lines, places of geopathic stress, underground water and their crossing places.

They may have been built to harness the energy of the fault lines, which give off high radiation levels. This can cause a shift in consciousness and perception. Certainly when visiting them today, time seems to stand still there, and meditation and inner journeying come easy. By spending time in these places, finding stillness and extending our awareness, we can perhaps intuit a sense of the past and its imprint on the present.

Caves

Find a cave you can go into and soak up the special atmosphere of being inside the Earth's living rock. Explore how this makes you feel and what it may awaken in you. Experience the damp air, the cold living stone and the darkness. Switch off your torch and soak up the dark. Take a candle and enjoy being in the cave in the flickering candlelight. Sing, tone and see what comes to you.

The more spectacular tourists caves are coming to the end of their season now and it is possible to book a private group visit and go into them with a group of friends. The acoustics in some of the big caverns are astonishing and it is worth doing some toning and chanting in them. You can request that the tour guide keeps the tourist chat to a minimum, and if you explain what you are doing, they are usually willing to stand aside and respectfully leave you to sit quietly, meditate, write poetry, sing or have a ceremony.

Commemorative Tree Planting

Trees can be planted to commemorate an event or a person. This can be part of a community event, or something you do to mark a personal connection. Trees need to be planted out between November and early March.

Often commemorative trees are fruit trees and can be planted to celebrate a marriage or anniversary, when a baby is born, to commemorate a teenager coming of age, for special anniversaries, any of the big 'O' birthdays or as a memorial for someone when they die.

When planting commemorative trees, take a moment to pause and say a few words before and after putting the tree in, dedicating the tree with due ceremony and fully honouring the reason for planting it.

Invite friends and family to bring spring water from different locations and special springs, and to each pour a libation on the earth beneath the tree and say a few words, or to bring a ribbon to tie into the tree. This helps each person to make a personal connection.

Planting Out Trees, page 97
Libations and Offerings, page 199

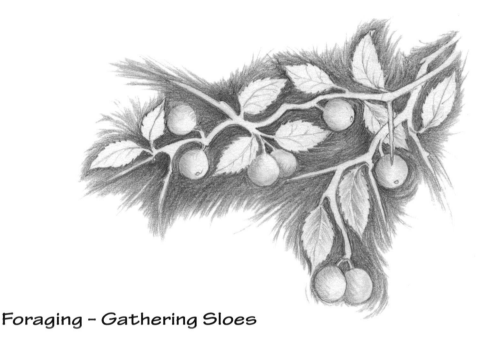

Foraging – Gathering Sloes

While you are out walking, keep an eye out for the blackthorn bushes and their ripening fruit, the sloes. They are found along the edges of fields and make thick impenetrable thickets, much loved by the birds and wildlife. A scratch from their thorns can easily turn septic so be careful when gathering sloes, which are traditionally picked after the first frosts have softened them. Make them into sloe gin and a dry red country wine.

Sloe Gin, page 84
Sloe Wine, page 85

SLOE INK
The juice makes a natural red dye and was once used as marking ink. Try drawing with it – use your fingers, a sharpened stick or the sharpened end of a feather for a really natural experience. Draw a picture of sloes with sloe juice!

THE WILD GARDENER

❋ No-dig Gardening ❋ Long Term Planning
❋ Growing Trees in Pots ❋ Growing Trees from Cuttings
❋ Guerrilla Gardening – Digging up and Planting Out

Often the day will look dark and dreary as I look out from inside, but the instant I am outside a miraculous transformation takes place and immediately I feel my spirits lift. I breathe deeply and feel instantly more alive. So this time of year wrap up warm and get out in the fresh air, and take every opportunity to soak up the natural light.

In this transition between autumn and winter there is plenty to do outside. Resist the urge to tidy up the plants too much though, especially around the wild edges. Let the vegetation die back naturally so that the plant's goodness returns to the soil and insects can find places to hibernate for the winter.

Pot up native biennials that have self-seeded and could be moved, planted out in the wild edges or given away.

See what spots near the house catch the low winter sun and move a bench there so that you can sit wrapped up warm with a cup of tea or breakfast, and enjoy some sunshine and watch the birds.

No-dig Gardening

At this time of year we see the earth covered by leaves and other decaying plant matter. What we don't see are the earthworms and small burrowing creatures transporting it all underground, along with the droppings and urine left by birds and other wildlife. We don't see the micro organisms and bacteria involved in breaking up the decaying plant matter and creating the rich and fertile humus that stores the nutrients for future plants. We don't see the bacteria and fungi creating food chains between the roots of plants. It is a delicate and intricate web of interrelationships and the argument for doing as little digging in the garden as possible, as digging quickly destroys what nature in her wild wisdom has created.

Pull out any plants that will not be useful as spring greens or medicine and spread a fine covering of compost, or horse manure over the bed. Let nature do the rest and your bed will be ready for planting in the spring.

Long Term Planning

Any big change in a garden layout needs to be planned in the winter months. This is part of the winter dreaming. While it is still fresh in your mind do a review of your gardening year, what worked and why. What changes would you like to make both in the garden and in yourself as a gardener?

Take into consideration what parts of the garden get the most sun and where gets the most shade. Which are your driest beds or wettest beds? What are your darkest least productive spots? What native plants could be grown there? Do you plan to have a wildlife area or a pond? Where do you like to sit? Where could you have a fire pit?

You can take advantage of being outside on dry sunny days and begin to draw up plans on paper. New beds can be marked out and covered with woollen carpet or cardboard to block out the light and suspend further growth, making digging out the roots easier in the spring.

Trees and hedge plants need to be moved and planted between now and early March.

Making a Pond, page 116

Growing Trees In Pots

Nuts and fruits such as acorns, hazelnuts, haws, wild plums, rowan, walnuts and chestnuts can be can be poked into labelled pots and left to grow. Cover with mesh if there is a danger of squirrels digging them up. Sprinkle other native seeds such as silver birch, elder and alder, into labelled pots.

Re-pot any trees you grew last year into bigger pots if they need it, giving them some fresh compost and generally giving them some attention and care. Make sure that the root collar – the point from which the roots grow – is just at the soil surface, and remove the bowls from under them now, as they dislike having their roots in cold or frozen water. If they are not too heavy, move them to a sunny spot for the winter.

You can also be creative with the trees as you repot them, raising them slightly each time so that you begin to expose roots. Put a slightly bigger stone under the roots each time you repot them. Young trees in pots can also be encouraged to bend and twist using string and wire. Be very gentle with the trees, only manipulating them a little at a time so as not cause them undue stress. These features will continue, as they become mature trees.

Sprinkle native plant seeds in with them or plant them up with native plants. This creates special partnerships, called guilds, which continue when you finally plant them out.

Creating Living Tree Sculptures, page 98
Collecting Tree Seeds, page 222

Growing Trees from Cuttings

ALDER, ELDER, HAZEL, HOLLY, WILLOW

This is an easy way to propagate new trees. Cuttings are best taken late autumn, early winter, and this is a great way to make use of some of your garden prunings.

1. Find a strong new shoot that is pencil thick and has many buds on it. Take the cutting just below a bud. Cut into 20cm (8in) lengths, with the bottom cut square to the twig just below a bud, and the top cut at an angle just above the top bud.

2. Store the cuttings by burying them in moist sand or compost and leave in cool dark place such as a shed or garage.

3. Between January and March plant the cuttings upright in the ground or in pots of moist compost, with about 5cm (2in) showing above ground.

4. By late spring the cuttings will be sprouting leaves. Keep the strongest shoot, and cut the rest off. Keep watered in dry weather and they will be ready for planting out in the autumn.

LEAF MOULD

This is a precious resource and it is worth gathering up leaves. Leaves can be bagged up and left to rot in their bags for a year and then added in layers to the compost bins. Native plants that previously would have grown in woodland also appreciate a dressing of leaf mould.

Guerrilla Gardening – Digging Up and Planting Out

Now is the time to look for young self-seeded native trees, either in your garden or any that are growing where they obviously have no chance of reaching maturity. You can spot them now as the vegetation begins to die back, and the young trees have enough leaves on them for identification. Mark with coloured ribbons or wool, with a colour code to identify each species and then dig them up over the next few months and move them to a better position.

If they are small then pot them into large plant pots with plenty of compost and nurture them until they are big enough to plant out in a year or two.

Native trees particularly suitable for rescuing and re-planting are elder, hawthorn, rowan, crab apple and hazel. All are very useful to the hedgerow forager and are all fairly small hedgerow trees.

Native perennials and first year native biennials can also be transplanted from your garden.

Guerrilla Gardening, pages 31, 98, 204

KITCHEN MEDICINE

❀ Digging Up and Drying Roots ❀ Making Root Tinctures

❀ Root Drinks – Dandelion and Burdock, Dandelion Coffee

❀ Blackthorn – Sloe Gin, Sloe Wine ❀ Simple Winter Posies

The garden is resting and this is the time to crack open the jars and bottles, enjoy the jam, pickles, and other delights you made in the summer and early autumn or wines from previous years. Your stores of medicines will help with winter colds and to boost up your immune system.

Digging Up and Drying Roots

Between November and March is the best time for digging up roots. They can be dug as part of the end of autumn garden tidy up.

Method

1. Scrub the dirt off them, dry with kitchen towel, chop them up, and put in brown paper bags.

2. Leave the roots to dry on the radiators or in a warm airy place, shaking them every few days.

3. When fully dry they can be stored in dark jars or fresh brown paper bags. (Don't forget to label them.)

4. They can be made into herbal teas by soaking them in cold water overnight and then bringing them to the boil and added to winter stews.

Decoction, page 44

Making Root Tinctures

DANDELION, VALERIAN
Now is the best time for making root tinctures when the energy of the plant has returned to the roots. Save any good roots you dig up when gardening.

Scrub them clean and cut into slices and make the tincture while they are still fresh. They can also be made from dried roots but soak them in a little water first. Use the soaking water as it is full of goodness.

For their herbal uses, see Plant Reference Guide, page 258, 276
Making Tinctures, page 46

Root Drinks

Root beers were once very popular. They are easy to make and ready in a week or two. They have the added advantage of imparting their herbal properties.

DANDELION AND BURDOCK BEER

Burdock roots are a prime blood purifier and detoxifier. It is an alkaline and helps counteract over-acidity. It stimulates the immune system to get rid of bacteria, toxins, viruses and tumour cells, strengthens the liver, kidneys, circulation, lungs, lymphatic and urinary systems, unblocking and detoxifying where ever they have become sluggish. It can be grown as a root vegetable but the roots are eaten in their first year only.

Dandelion roots are a prime liver and lymph tonic, and a good digestive tonic.

Method
1. Scrub two large dandelion roots and two large burdock roots.

2. Chop them into a pan with 2.25 litres (4 pints) of water. Boil for half an hour.

3. In another pan, gently dissolve one pound of sugar in four pints of water with 2 tablespoons of black treacle and the juice of a lemon.

4. Strain off the roots, mix the two liquids together and leave to go tepid.

5. Then add an ounce of yeast mixed to a paste with warm water.

6. Leave to ferment in a covered bucket for three to four days, then bottle. Ready to drink after 1 week.

DANDELION COFFEE

Worth saving are any of the big roots you dig up to make into dandelion coffee. It is easy to make, delicious to drink, and of course holds all the beneficial properties of dandelion root.

Method

1. Dig plants up when the soil is wet so that the long roots slide out easily. Scrub them clean and then leave them to dry out somewhere warm for a couple of days.

2. Slice them and chop them finely or rough chop in a food processor.

3. Spread out on a baking tray and roast for 1 or 2 hours on a medium to high oven with the door open. The size of the pieces and the level of roast is a matter of personal taste.

4. When cool grind them in a coffee grinder and store in a dark jar.

Blackthorn (*Prunus spinosa*)

Making sloe gin is one of those end-of-year delights as we say goodbye to the old year and give thanks for its rich harvest.

SLOE GIN

Traditionally wait until after the first frost has softened the sloes. You can also pick them before and put them in the freezer to mimic nature.

1. Fill one-third of a wide-necked jar with sloes that have been pricked.

2. Make it up to half full with organic sugar and fill to the top with a good quality gin.

3. Shake daily for 3 months and watch the gin turn deep red.

4. Strain off the fruit, but do not squeeze. Rebottle, keeping some for the Solstice and some to save for 1 year for an improved flavour.

5. Rather than throw the gin soaked fruit away, cut the flesh from the stones and add to melted chocolate or chocolate cake!

SLOE WINE

> 1.35kg (3lb) sloes
> 1kg (2.2lb) sugar
> 2 oranges
> 4 litres (1 gallon) water
> 1 teaspoon yeast

1. Boil the sloes in half the water for 30 minutes, crushing them with a wooden spoon to break the skins and release the juice.

2. Pour to a clean bucket with the rest of the boiled water, the peel and juice of the oranges, cover and leave for three days, stirring every day.

3. Strain and bring to the boil with the sugar until the sugar is dissolved.

4. Let the liquid cool to lukewarm, stir in the yeast and then pour into a demijohn.

5. Fit an air lock and leave in a warm place until it stops fermenting.

6. Siphon off into wine bottles, cork and label.
   Wait for a year before drinking.

Simple Winter Posies

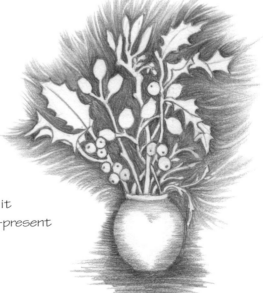

Pick a small vase of beautiful things from the garden such as herbs, seed heads, twigs, evergreens and the last of the flowers and bring them into the kitchen. Renew it frequently. There is always something to find and to celebrate in the garden and it means that the outdoors is an ever-present inspiration in your home.

SEASONAL CELEBRATIONS

❋ Samhain

❋ Making an End of Year Headdress or Mask

❋ Making Elder Beads

The days are short now and we sense the wild edges of winter creeping in. This is the beginning of the deepest darkest part of the year. We recognise our own need to rest now, like the Earth, to slow down and adjust to a new set of conditions. It is time to finally let go of the old year, to follow the urge to withdraw, to remember who we are on the inside, reflect on the old year and dream the seeds of the future we wish to see happen.

Welcome these dark days as an opportunity to shift your focus from achieving and doing, to reflecting and assimilating all that comes to rest in you now.

Samhain
End of October – Beginning of November

The festival of Samhain (pronounced sow-ein), is one of the great fire festivals of our ancient past, affirming regeneration and rebirth in the midst of endings and darkness. Celebrated on 31st October or the nearest dark moon, and overlaid by the church as All Hallows Eve, Halloween.

In the Celtic tradition Samhain was recognised as a special time of year. It is a time when the veil between the worlds is thin, when we can seek communication with other realms that lie along side of ours or within ourselves. The Celts called this the Otherworld. We can push the wild edges of our perceptions and assumptions, to seek out what truths this may hold for us.

This is an opportunity to move from the popular myth that the dark is a place to fear and choose to see the dark as a place of renewal and regeneration. When we see the dark of the year as part of our own cycle and needs, we recognise that we can, like the Earth, make time to rest now, send down our roots, and strengthen ourselves on the inside.

The Earth teaches us that everything in nature is cyclic – death will eventually lead to rebirth. But first like the Earth, we must have a period of rest, gather the seeds of our future intentions and nurture them in our dark and fertile imaginations. These seeds and future visions will grow within us, and as part of the interconnected web of life they will become fertile in ways we could never imagine for ourselves.

Samhain is a celebration of all that has finished and ended, the seasonal end of the old year. We are called upon to let our old selves die so that we can expand and grow into new parts of ourselves.

This endless cycle of change is healthy and necessary, bringing renewal of understanding, renewal of cells and regeneration from within. It is an opportunity for us to honour what has finished and ended, so that when the time comes, we are ready for the new beginnings that present themselves.

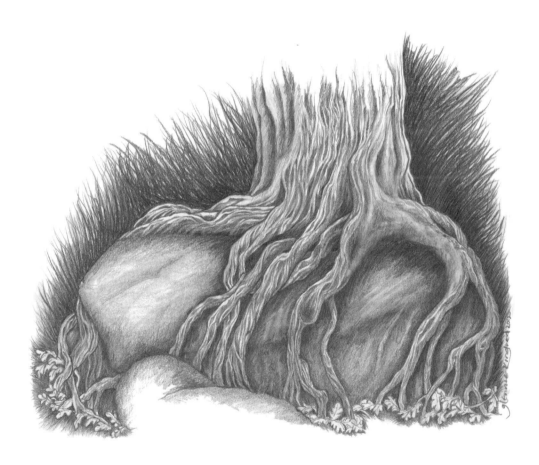

SAMHAIN CELEBRATIONS

Included here are some ideas for connecting to the Earth, the seasonal energy, and your inner wisdom at this time. Choose a couple of things to do, and be open to your own spontaneous inspirations of the moment.

For insights and overview about co-creating seasonal gatherings, see page 66

• Gather with friends for a Samhain celebration. Each bring seasonal food to share, made from roots, the last of the vegetables from the garden, apples or dried fruit and berries. Share preserves, fruit cordials and last years berry wines.

• If celebrating on your own then make yourself special seasonal food and treats!

• Fire is important, so if possible have a fire outside. If this isn't possible then fill a large wide bowl with earth or sand and light candles at the centre of the gathering circle.

• Create a central focus of colourful autumn leaves, nuts, seed and seed-heads, and give thanks for the end of the Earth's growth cycle and the seeds that ensure it will continue.

• Make some time at the beginning of the celebration for reflection and meditation. Sit and stare into the fire or candle flames and remember the old year. Reflect upon the joys you experienced, as well as the difficulties. Look for the hidden blessings that they may hold. Remember all the special places that you visited in this beautiful land of ours, and your experiences there. Write them down in your journal and if gathered with others, share the highlights and your insights.

• Write down what you leave behind in the old year, what is no longer helpful to you. Include old beliefs and old attitudes that dampen your life force and the life force of the Earth. Write on pieces of pager and burn them in the fire if you are outside. If you are inside then light them from the candles and put them in a lidded pot to finish burning. Say anything you need to say as you burn them. The burnt remains can be taken outside and put back on the earth or buried later.

• Each throw a stick or a dead leaf in the fire to represent what you let go of. Name them out loud to give weight to your resolve. Later write about your feelings about this in your journal.

• Each light a candle and make a pledge to the Earth to be part of her human support system. Pledge to give something back, such as time and energy to help her, and pledge to stop doing the things that are not helping her ecosystem to repair. Name these in sacred space.

• Light a candle for yourself. Be peaceful and at rest with yourself. Promise to nurture yourself in the dark. Name ways that you might do this. What restful things will you do this winter? What will fill you with happiness? What will help you move forwards?

• Resolve to keep moving into a holistic consciousness and not stay stuck in old separation thinking patterns. Look for where you have changed your thinking and have become more connected to the Earth this last year. Look for the triggers that help you to create connection. Share these insights with each other.

• Find ways to become more integrated in your local communities this winter. What groups could you join? What groups that already exist could you support? What new group could you set up? Be prepared to communicate, to accept and be open with each other, beyond judgment, beyond 'Us and Them', to embrace the 'We' of our common humanity. Share your ideas and see who else is interested.

• This is the season of remembrance, a time to remember our ancestors and those who have died, including people we didn't know personally but have touched our lives. Invite everyone to bring photos of them. Make a special Ancestors Shrine. Light candles for them. Share your thoughts with each other.

• There are a lot of little deaths in our lives, losses, things we will never get back. Take a moment to name these losses and then look for the positive gifts they might hold. Light candles for these things and find peace in reflective silence and your personal philosophy.

• Pass round a bowl of acorns, hazel nuts, haws or rowan berries. Take one to represent each gift or lesson you feel you have gained this year. Name them and plant them in a pot of earth to grow. Label the pot and decorate by wrapping it in material and coloured wool. Put the pot outside without a bowl under it, and you might be rewarded by a tree shoot in the spring.

• As we go into the winter, ask yourself: What do I need to do to look after myself and help myself to regenerate in the dark?

• What are your Visions of Hope for the future? Write in your journal and share your thoughts, feelings and insights with each other. All our actions make a difference. What can you do to help this to happen?

• What do you want to nurture in the dark? Write your thoughts on pieces of silver birch bark or card cut into hearts or leaves. With a large-eyed needle and embroidery thread, hang them up or make into a simple mobile to delight and remind you.

Make An End Of Year Headdress or Mask

Masks and headdresses made from the last of the vegetation of the old year are very traditional at Samhain.

1. Use pliable stems of dogwood, ivy, honeysuckle or willow to create an initial circlet to fit the head or the frame of a mask shape to fit the face, and then weave or tie in autumn leaves, berries and seed heads. Use a natural thread to help tie the stems in place.

2. Wear it at the beginning of the celebration to honour the old year. It can then be burnt in the fire at some point, to represent what you let go of, from the old year, in order to move forwards. Name these as you throw it in the fire.

3. Alternatively return it to the Earth with your thanks to compost down. Something may grow from the seeds that were in it! With this in mind, you might like to lay it on a pot of earth outside your door.

Make Elder Beads

Elder represents the power of the regenerative life force, and reminds us that in every ending there is always a new beginning. Its herbal action encourages us to throw off congestion and stuck energy. Small elder branches, about 2cm (¾in) in diameter, can be cut and sawn into beads. Respect the tree and ask first. If you sense you are not welcome to cut the branch, then ask another tree. Elder, more than any other native tree, has a lot of folklore surrounding the respect due to the tree before cutting it.

1. Saw the stem into small pieces between one and 2cm (¾in) in length.

2. Inside the stem is a soft pith, which can easily be poked out with a nail, or bradawl. This makes a natural bead.

3. The bark can be shaved off with a penknife and then sanded down. As you peel the bark from the bead, peel off what you let go of in your life and no longer need. Burn the parings and speak out what you leave behind.

4. Elder has a beautiful yellow oily close-grained wood, which polishes up well with fine sandpaper. Any herbal oils you have made during the year can be used to feed the wood and add to your intention and resolve.

5. Thread the bead onto leather thread or thin elastic to make a necklace or bracelet. Add other beads or shells or tie on coloured threads to represent the threads of new ideas you take into the dark to incubate.

6. Create a special ceremonial moment to honour the moment and say what your beads mean to you.

Elder beads can also used like a wooden toggle for fastening clothing, bags and pouches.

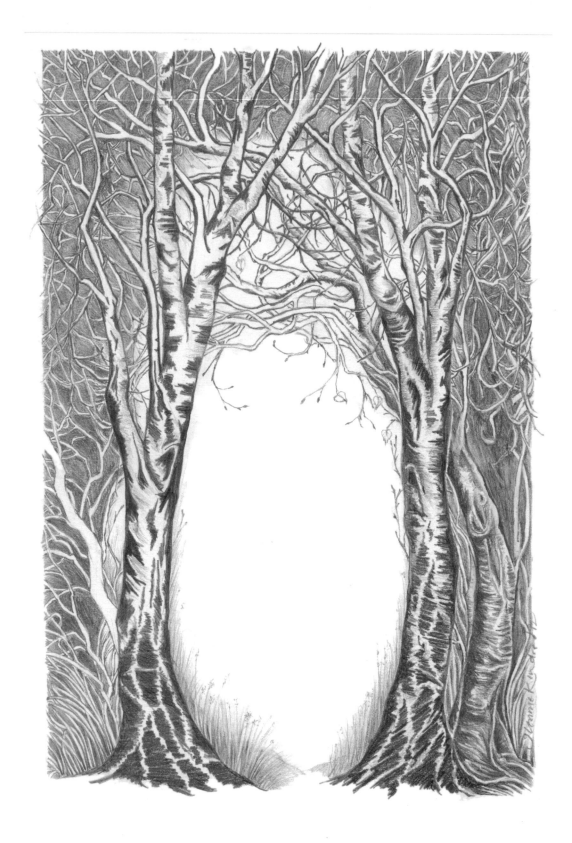

WINTER'S
wild edge

December into January

The Earth is resting now and if we can, we must slow down and rest too. It is a good time to settle back into our local environment and appreciate the land and the friends and neighbours we have around us. Winter brings shortness of daylight and above ground there is very little growth, but below the surface roots are growing, bringing stability and strength to the plants and trees that will support their future growth.

The dark of the winter gives us the opportunity to connect to what lies within us, so that we too grow strong roots, which will strengthen us on the inside and bring greater stability. Use this time to rest, to reflect and dream in the dark. Make time for study, reading, creative projects, art, music, writing, musing and meditation. These things help us to expand inwards and experience this vital edge of our whole selves.

Learn from the Earth. Look at how you can live your life with an awareness of the interconnectedness of all things. Everything we do and everything we say, think and feel, ripples out into the web of life around us, as well as into our bodies and consciousness, affecting our health and the health of our environment. Use the winter to vision the future you want for yourself and for the Earth. Plan how you will make changes in your life and lifestyle to help this happen.

OUT ON THE LAND

❁ Transition Into a New Cycle

❁ Winter Walking

❁ Visiting Trees

❁ Walking with Friends

Don't be put off by wild weather days, wrap up warm and enjoy wild walks in the rain and mists, appreciating the delicate subtle beauty of the winter landscape. Make the most of sunny days. Celebrate all the elements and our seasonal cycle as part of the richness of life and the Earth's beautiful diversity. Getting out in the fresh air helps revive our spirits and it is always much brighter outside than it appears from the inside.

This is the point in the Earth's cycle when the days are at their shortest and the nights are at their longest. The Winter Solstice marks this most extreme point in the year's cycle, and from here the days will begin to lengthen again. Even though there are still many winter days to come, we experience this as a turning point.

Transition Into a New Cycle

On your walks look for somewhere you could use a natural feature to use to mark your transition into the new cycle. It doesn't have to be exactly at the Solstice, just sometime around this time. Look for a natural feature in the landscape such as an archway created by two trees, a row of trees to walk through, or a cleft in a rock to squeeze through.

Pause at the threshold and gather into your heart all that has moved you in the last 6 months since the Summer Solstice. As you step through the archway, name your wishes for the new cycle about to begin. Picture them happening and already in motion. You could also go through twice, once to let go of what you leave behind in the old cycle and a second time to make an intention, a promise or pledge to yourself and to the Earth.

Thresholds, Doorways and Archways, page 64

Winter Walking

Winter walking is invigorating, gets our circulation going, and balances our tendency to hide indoors at this time of year. Remember what a treat it is to be out in the wild weather, wrap up warm and immediately you will feel the benefit as soon as you step outside.

Make the most of blue-sky days, frosty mornings, hoarfrost on the trees and days of pale winter sunshine and fill your eyes and hearts with wonder for the beauty of the Earth.

Visiting places in the winter is one of my great joys. Chances are you will not meet anyone else and you will be able to soak up the atmosphere of a place without interruption. Look at maps of your locality, old and new. Discover the places you don't know, especially seeking out the tumulus hills, any little known stone circles, burial mounds or the hill forts of our long distant past. You may well sense the special energy these special hills still hold. Look for other significant hills in the landscape that they may be linked to.

Visiting Trees

Trees provide us with shelter from the winds and often a dry place to sit and watch the world go by. Trees help us to slow down and appreciate deeper levels of connection to the Earth. Remember there is as much tree below the ground as above, and imagine their deep roots interweaving and growing beneath the surface, claiming their space and anchoring these great beings to the Earth.

When out walking in the woods, find a special tree on high ground that you can climb up into and make your 'Lookout tree'. Enjoy the elevated views across the woods and the land. Let yourself daydream a while and see what rises to the surface from the depths of you.

Walking with Friends

Get out on the land with friends and make an agreement between you that you will go out on your chosen day whatever the weather. Celebrating wild weather days is contagious and we can all help each other to find out that we actually like them!

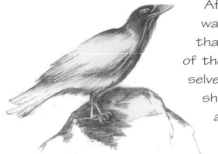

After initial chats and catch-ups, agree to walk in silence for some part of the walk, so that each can become absorbed in the wonders of the natural world and have space for themselves. Agree that if you do speak it is only to share your experiences of the natural world around you.

At this time of year plan a route that will include a village pub for lunch and warming up.

THE WILD GARDENER

❀ Looking After the Birds ❀ Planting Out Trees
❀ Making Living Tree Sculptures
❀ Guerrilla Gardening – Finding Homes For Native Trees

It is so good to get out in the garden in the winter, breathe some fresh air and see how things are getting on. Quickly it becomes obvious that life continues and everywhere there are signs of new life emerging. Many of the native plants are already popping up and clusters of small new leaves are growing at the heart of many of the perennials. If edible, these can be picked and eaten. Buds are beginning to form on some of the trees and the first bulbs are pushing through the dark wet earth.

Looking After the Birds

Birds help us to connect to the wild edges of the natural world. In the winter we can provide food for them to see them through the worst of the winter weather and in return we have the pleasure of watching them and getting to know them better.

Place bird feeders near the house and out of reach of cats, where you can observe the birds without disturbing them. Provide them with a wide shallow bowl of water for drinking and bathing in. When the weather freezes make sure it is kept ice-free. Feeding takes a lot of their time and energy when it is cold, so try to avoid disturbing them when they are feeding.

Make an undercover bird table on a post and scatter crumbs and seeds here for robins, dunnocks and wrens.

Sunflower heads, fat balls, and a bird feeders of seed mixtures and peanuts will encourage greenfinches, chaffinches, bullfinches, blue tits, great tits, coal tits and sparrows.

Blackbirds and thrushes, fieldfares and redwings will come into the garden to eat old bruised apples and apple cores. We throw ours under our fruit trees and this encourages them to forage in the leaf-fall and eat up fruit tree pest larvae, slugs and snails.

Planting Out Trees

Trees need to be planted out or moved between November and March while the sap is down and while roots can grow and get established before the sap rises.

1. Water the tree well before planting out.

2. Dig a hole big enough for the root bowl and big enough for the tree to spread its roots. Throw in a bucket of compost or well-rotted horse manure and water in the hole before planting the tree.

3. Make sure that the root collar – the point from which the roots grow – is just at the soil surface unless you have been raising the tree to have some exposed roots showing.

4. Firm the soil well down around the base of the tree and water again.

5. Cut some sturdy straight sticks from ash or hazel to use as a stake and add a tree guard for added protection.

6. Keep an eye on the tree for the first year, keep grasses away from its base and water if the weather is dry.

Growing Trees in Pots, page 79

Creating Living Tree Sculptures

A semi circle of small trees can be planted to create living dens, hideaways and arbours. Both willow and hazel saplings are good for this but other saplings also work. It depends on the structure being created. The young whips can be pulled over, bent into shape, woven and tied to create places to sit in and places for children to play in. They have to be regularly worked on especially in their early stages to get the right shape, and newly grown sprigs need to be woven in regularly. Once a good shape has been established, keep it regularly trimmed during the summer to encourage denser foliage to keep out the rain.

Also consider planting two or three trees of the same species together in a pot and weaving their trunks together while they are still pliant and young. They always want to untie themselves so you will need to keep an eye on them. They can also be grafted together by splicing them where you want them to join and wrapping the join with string or cling film for a season while they heal.

Living hazel seats and benches can also be created in this way. It takes constant attention to get a good shape, selecting the branches that will be the seat, and the back, pruning off unwanted branches and grafting the joints well. Pruning helps direct the growth into the desired shape. A cut above a leaf or node can help direct the tree to grow where you want it to grow. If a leaf points to the right, then cut above the leaf to produce new growth that will grow to the right. Similarly, a cut above a leaf pointing to the left, produces new growth that grows to the left.

Growing a chair takes many years and there is no guarantee of success, but it is an interesting project to attempt. John Krubsack famously grew chairs in the early 1900s and there are some wonderful photos of him sitting in his chairs, both when they were still growing and later after they were cut.

Resources, page 281

Guerrilla Gardening – Finding Homes For Native Trees

If your trees in pots have got to a good size, it may be time to find places to plant them out. This must be done between November and early March. If you have land this is easy; if not, like me, then creative ways have to be found!

Give them to friends, community projects and to anyone who has land and is happy to have more trees, and wants to build up mixed hedgerows or replace hedgerows that may have been taken out in the past. These will provide places for the birds to nest and other wildlife to live, and creates new wild edges for native plants to grow along. Planting the nut and fruit bearing native trees will provide more foraging opportunities for the future. Particularly good to plant out are elder, hawthorn, rowan and hazel.

Public places, such as schools, colleges, churchyards, parks, and hospitals, often have space for trees and would welcome you asking them.

Most native trees can be used for creating hedges for gardens and allotments, making windbreaks and adding to the ecodiversity. Ash, willow and hazel can be selectively coppiced to provide the gardener with an endless supply of straight sticks for bean poles and tying up plants.

It may also involve a bit of guerrilla gardening, by planting them out in places that would benefit from a tree or two, such as playgrounds, along walkways and trails, by rivers, on roadsides and verges, in towns, along hedgerows, canal sides, up on the moors, along woodland edges and on the edge of any forgotten piece of land.

When planting out trees remember the size that the tree will eventually become and consider if it has enough space to grow and if the type and size of the tree is appropriate there. Trees in more confined places will be more stunted, and grow more slowly.

Add a bucket of compost at the bottom of the hole before planting the tree and water well. Bang in a stake and protect with a tree guard and chances are they will be treated as if they are meant to be there. Keep an eye on them for their first year, until their roots get established and take bottles of water to water them if the weather is dry.

Growing Trees in Pots, page 79
Planting Out Trees, page 97

KITCHEN MEDICINE

❀ Boosting Your Immune System

❀ Making Your Own Cough Medicine

❀ Herbal Baths and Footbaths ❀ Make Time to Rest

❀ Voluntary Simplicity

The winter is time for resting, regenerating and relaxing. Be gentle with yourself. Love yourself. Do what makes you happy! Nourish yourself with good home cooked food, homemade cakes and other delights. Use all the wonderful things you have carefully stored and preserved during the autumn.

Now we reap the benefits of all the herbs we have picked, dried, made into tinctures or elixirs during the summer months. Each year, as your knowledge and passion for the herbs grows, there are always more you wish you had, and a resolve to grow or collect more of a certain herb you want to use in the winter. Make notes of these and find places where you can order native plant seeds. Dried herbs can be ordered and sent through the post if you have run out of the herbs you find you need.

Resources, page 281

Boosting Your Immune System

Elderberry tincture or elixir is essential to take at this time of the year for colds, congestion and coughs and to boost the immune system. Take a teaspoonful daily in a glass of water to boost up the immune system and help prevent colds. At the first sign of a sore throat, take a teaspoonful of elderberry tincture or syrup three times a day.

If you didn't manage to collect elderberries in the autumn, buy dried elderberries. Make the tincture or elixir in the usual way, leaving a little extra room in the jar for the elderberries to swell. Drink hot elderberry wine to bring out a fever and clear the chest of congestion.

You can't beat raw garlic for fighting off infections and boosting the immune system. Chop it finely and sprinkle over the tops of soups or any savoury dish just before serving, to get your daily dose. Whizz into fruit smoothies (a lot more delicious than it sounds!).

Making Tinctures, page 46
Making Elixirs, page 48
Elderberry Wine, page 234
Herb Suppliers, page 283

Making Your Own Cough Medicine

Ribbed Plantain (*Plantago lanceolata*) is very abundant this time of year and can be found growing everywhere. It is a prime remedy for coughs and can be made into a herbal infusion or a herbal honey. Honey's antibacterial quality rapidly clears infection and taken with or without the herbs will help a cough or sore throat.

If you have dried any of the following herbs in the summer then add them to the herbal honey cough mixture: coltsfoot, chickweed, dandelion, elderflowers or berries, mullein flowers or leaves, nettles, thyme, or violets. Leave the honey soaked herbs for a few days to steep and keep topping up with more plants and honey.

Honey elixirs can be quickly made using tinctures and honey. They are ideal for taking out in your pocket but are for adults only because of the brandy.

Method 2, Making Honey Elixirs, page 49
Making Herbal Honeys, page 51

Herbal Baths and Footbaths

Treat yourself to a relaxing herbal bath or soak your feet in a herbal foot bath. The herbs are absorbed easily through the skin in the hot water. By using the herbs you dried in the summer you are bringing them into your life and your experience of them grows. They become part of what you do and it keeps the connection with the plants through the winter.

Make a hot herbal infusion from your stores of dried herbs, cover and infuse for 10 minutes before pouring in the bath or a washing up bowl for a footbath.

Use any of the following native plants or any combination of these:

To Relax and Restore

Make an infusion of vervain, hawthorn flowers or leaves, rose petals, cowslips, St Johns wort.

Before Bed to Bring Relaxed Sleep

Make an infusion of hops, cowslip, elderflowers, hawthorn flowers, red clover, violets, thyme or chamomile.

For Tired and Painful Muscles

Dandelion flowers and leaves, hops, St Johns wort, violet, meadowsweet or any combination of these.

As a General Tonic

Cleavers, cowslips, dandelion, nettle, vervain or any combination of these.

For Colds, Flu or Fever

Elderflowers, mint, vervain, yarrow or any combination of these.

Add some of your aromatic kitchen herbs to any bath mix such as lavender, chamomile or borage, to bring relaxation or rosemary to stimulate, revitalise and get your circulation going.

Absorbing Herbs Through the Skin, page 52
Infusions, page 44
Making Bath Bags, page 206

Make Time to Rest

Many illnesses are born out of stress and forgetting to weave in periods of rest. They are often a call to stop and do nothing, which is why it is often a relief to have a few days in bed when we are ill. If you don't get enough quality rest time, look at where you need to make changes in your lifestyle so that it is less stressful, and establish new patterns into your daily routine.

Ask friends to help you if you need some extra help. Friends are always willing to help each other, but most of us forget to ask them. Gift yourself quality rest time, book a massage, or do more of whatever you do that makes you happy.

Most importantly, get outside for frequent walks in beautiful places.

When you feel stressed or off centre, remember to breathe slowly and send your roots deep down into the earth below you. Picture yourself becoming anchored by your roots. Rest in the dark nurturing stillness.

Find your joyful connection to the simple pleasures of life such as cooking, simple craftwork, making fires and being with friends and family. Make someone a cake, or a meal and share some of your autumn preserves.

Voluntary Simplicity

Live lightly on the Earth. Look for ways to simplify your lifestyle that will make you happy and the Earth a better place. Have a good clearout, and clutter-clear your home-space. Look for where you are encumbered by possessions or past achievements. Be open to self-imposed change. Let go of your old baggage. What weighs you down and blocks your joy? Create space for future possibilities to happen. Affirm your willingness to begin the new when the time is right.

SEASONAL CELEBRATIONS

❀ Winter Solstice

❀ Traditional Native Evergreens

❀ Make a Solstice Bush

❀ Make a Holly Touchwood

Midwinter is the darkest time of the year, and it is good to make peace with this and to see it as a vital part of the balance of life. Enjoy peaceful days and 'Go Slow' days. Shut down, withdraw and rest in the dark of the year. Now we begin to deepen the understanding and insights we have gained in this reflective time. Gradually we begin to see what our new seeds may be, and strengthen and consolidate what we would like to take forward into the new outer-growth cycle when it comes.

Winter Solstice
20th – 23rd December

The sun has reached its most southern extreme for the year, rising in the extreme south east and setting in the extreme south west. The darkness has reached its height. This is the longest day and shortest night of the year in the Northern Hemisphere. From this point onwards the days will begin to lengthen and eventually warmth will return to the land.

Winter Solstice, like Summer Solstice, is a moment of pause between two cycles, a moment of transition that can be held and savoured, a doorway, an opening, a place on the edge, when we can stop our busy lives and take a moment to experience this edge between these two great cycles of the year. We can look back on our journey since the Summer Solstice, to acknowledge what we have completed in this cycle, what we have experienced and what wisdom we have gained. It is also a moment to look forward, to name the new seeds and intentions we wish to take into the next cycle.

WINTER SOLSTICE CELEBRATIONS

Included here are some ideas for connecting to the Earth, the seasonal energy, and your inner wisdom. Choose a couple of things to do, and be open to your own spontaneous inspirations of the moment.

For insights and overview about co-creating seasonal gatherings, see page 66

For insights and overview about co-creating seasonal gatherings, see page 66

• In the age-old tradition, go out early on this special morning, whatever the weather. Find somewhere to watch the Solstice sunrise and enjoy whatever the dawn brings. Look back on the year you have just had and reflect on the wisdom you gained from it. Then look forwards, taking into your heart the most positive, the most loving, the most inspirational future you could wish for yourself and the Earth.

• Make an arrangement with friends to meet before dawn and walk to a high point that faces south east, and has a long view to the horizon. Make connection to Earth and affirm how you will live your life with an increased awareness of the Earth's needs. Afterwards go back to someone's house for a shared breakfast.

• If possible spend the rest of the day together, at someone's house or hire a hall for a Winter Solstice gathering. Winter Solstice is an opportunity to gather with friends in your community, to be loving and generous, to share abundance, to celebrate community and to share our hopes for the new cycle. Ask everyone to bring seasonal food to share, drums and percussion, a community gift (something to offer to the day such as a performance, a game, a song etc) and a small wrapped gift for the giveaway basket – something that you wish to give away or have made. Have clearly labelled separate baskets for adults and children.

Drum, dance, feast and entertain each other throughout the day. At some point gather in a circle, give thanks to the Earth that sustains us. Count your blessings and give thanks for your abundance and friendships. Pass round the giveaway basket so each takes a present.

• If it is possible, light a fire outside, however briefly. If this is not possible then fill a large dish with sand and light lots of candles. Share stories round the fire or the candle cluster. There is nothing more magical than sitting together around living flame. Children become calm and everyone becomes peaceful and connected.

• If indoors, decorate the centre of the room with evergreens. As you cut them, connect to the life force of the land and thank the trees and bushes for their gift. Remember the birds will need the berries, so don't over pick.

• Create a centre-piece of evergreens and a large bowl of soil or compost. Gather in a circle around this. Light a central candle with a heartfelt dedication. Switch off the lights so that the single flame at the centre is the only light. Have a quiet few minutes and lose yourself as you stare at the single candle flame. Breathe deeply in the darkness and the stillness. Switch off your busy mind, keep focused on the flame, and rest in the dark.

Place a basket of candles next to it. Invite everyone to light a candle for the return of the light, for the Earth or what you wish to give thanks for. Each say out loud what ever comes to you as you do this. As each lights their candle, the room gradually fills with light.

• Create time to reflect on your personal year. What has made you happy and what has made you sad? What lessons have been learnt? What will grow out of these lessons and this old cycle? What do you want to see happen in the new year to come? Write in your journal and share with each other.

If this is a group that meets regularly together, reflect on your year together as a group and take it in turns to share your review of the year.

• It is important that we take good energy with us into the new cycle. Ask yourself what sustains and nurtures you? Write this down in your journal and share with the rest of the group. What negative aspects of yourself do you leave behind in the old year? What positive qualities do you want to take with you? Write in your journal and share with each other. From the review, begin to form the seeds of your new intentions for the new cycle.

• In the coming cycle what do you choose to put your energy into? In what way can you make a positive difference? How can you help the Earth? What seeds can you now begin to sow that will help to unite your needs with the Earth's needs? Each take a night-light and as you light it, speak out your new intentions. Fire up what you want for the Earth and yourself. Place them in small dishes around the central shrine.

• What self-imposed limitations stop you visioning the most exciting, most expansive, most healing possibilities for your new seeds? What limits the flow or blocks your new intentions? Share your insights in pairs and write them down in your journal. Then spend some time helping each other to create a positive affirmation that will bring about changing this. Each step into the circle and speak out their positive affirmation. Everyone drum and cheer!

• Fill your glasses with a hot spicy fruit cup made from the fruits of the Earth and invite everyone to raise their glasses and toast the Earth, and any new intentions you have made to help her. Raise your glasses and toast the new cycle to come, what you wish to welcome in and the things you value in each other.

• Winter is a time for dreaming and visioning the future. Vision a future of environmental and social justice and affirm your support for this with everything you buy, consume and do. Affirm daily that you always make conscious choices that support this. Give thanks to the Earth, for the abundance of food we have in this country. Vision a future of fair shares for all, a future where we no longer waste food but share it amongst those who need it.

When people stand together in a just cause we can change what happens next. Each light three candles or hang three ribbons in the trees as you make three new intentions to help the environment and the Earth.

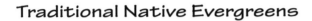

• Give thanks for all the Earth's resources that make our present lives possible and vision a future of renewable sustainable energy systems that do not harm the Earth or threaten our lives. Write in your journal your 'Visions of Hope' for the new year. What could you do to help them manifest? Light a candle and name your new year intentions.

Traditional Native Evergreens

Traditionally, native evergreens would have been bought in to decorate the houses to symbolically affirm life in the dark of the year. See if you can intuit for yourself what their symbolic significance is as you spend a little time with each of the trees and plants before cutting them. Traditionally these would have been holly, ivy, mistletoe, pine and yew.

N.B. Yew is poisonous so do not bring in around children.

Don't cut too many of the berried twigs as the birds will need them for their food. Use what berried twigs you do cut to the greatest effect.

MAKE AN EVERGREEN CENTREPIECE

Half fill a wide dish with water. Place a large wide-bottomed candle at the centre and arrange various evergreens around it with their ends in the water. Light the candle every day with wishes and affirmations. When the festive season is over, cut off any usable wood to whittle and return the rest of the vegetation to the Earth with your thanks.

Make a Simple Wheel of the Year Door Wreath

Weave fine long twigs of willow, ivy, honeysuckle and any other flexible plant stems into a circle and then poke and tie in evergreens with thin florists wire. Afterwards return it to the Earth with thanks.

Make an Evergreen Headdress

Using long whips of willow, ivy or dogwood, make a circlet to fit your head. Then poke and tie in evergreens and wear it at your Solstice celebration. Afterwards return it to the Earth with thanks.

Make a Headdress, pages 90, 172

Make A Solstice Bush

Rather than cut down a tree, cut twigs from various evergreen trees and bushes, or simple bare branches, and arrange in a vase, large pot or bucket. This can be wrapped up with coloured paper or material and wrapped round with ribbon or wool. Fill with water. If they are large heavy twigs then also add stones to the bucket to give it weight. Keep checking the water levels as twigs are thirsty. Being indoors the buds on the bare branches will swell and eventually leaf. If you cut from trees or bushes that have blossom in the spring, then the blossom will come out sometime in January. Save some of the cutting back in the garden for this moment and enjoy them as your Solstice bush.

Ask family, friends and visitors to tie on ribbons to represent their new hopes and wishes for the future. Have a small basket of cut ribbons ready for this.

Make A Holly Touchwood

A touchwood is a small piece of wood that you keep in your pocket to remind you of an intention made or a focus you wish to keep.

Our native holly tree remains green throughout the winter and is a potent reminder of the power of the life force. Holly grows straight and reminds us to set clear directions for ourselves so that we move forward with clarity.

Holly wood is white and fine grained. It will sand up with fine sandpaper to look like bone. Get down to the bare bones of what saps and depletes your life force, as you take off the bark with a penknife. As you take off the bark imagine yourself unburdened by these things. Burn the peelings in a fire or candle, and say out loud in the present tense, that you leave… (name them)… behind in the old year.

Now you have revealed the beautiful white wood inside. Take a moment to gather to yourself what strengthens your life force and resolve to do more of this in the new year.

Hold these in your heart as you sand the piece of holly, first with rough sandpaper, then with medium, and then with fine and finally with extra fine.

Make a clear statement of intention, write it in your journal and if you are with others, share this with the group.

Keep the holly touchwood in your pocket as a reminder of the things that energise your life force and your intended new directions.

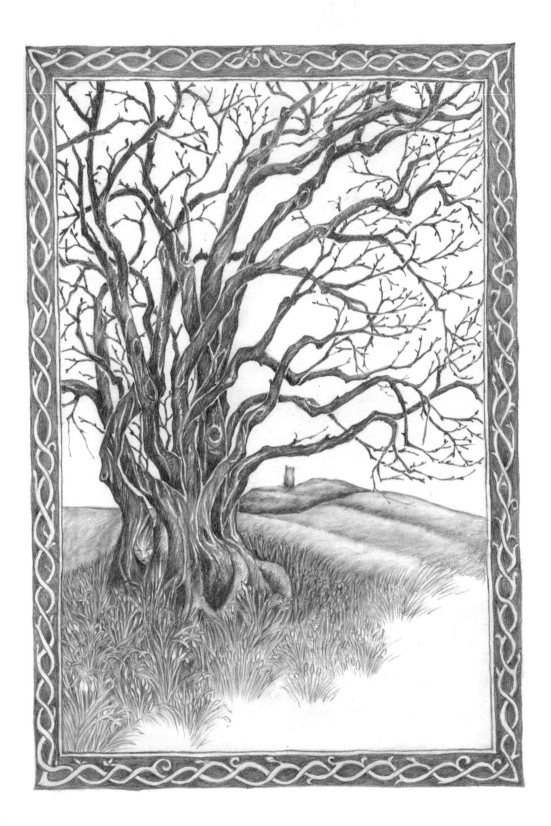

on the edge of
SPRING

January into February

The old year has died but within the decay there are signs of new life growing. The first bright green shoots of the spring bulbs are poking through the soil. Hazel catkins glow in the welcome sunlight and everywhere there is the feeling that life is stirring. Seen from a distance, some of the native trees have taken on a coloured hue, caused by the gentle swelling of their buds, faint at first, but increasing as the increase in the days length begins to influence the plants. There is a sense of rebirth in the air, of new beginnings waiting for their right time to come.

With this Earth-awakening comes new opportunities to make simple but life-changing shifts in our lifestyles and thinking patterns. Living more sustainably and with greater awareness of the Earth is something we can no longer ignore. The time for dreaming is over. The time for action begins. We do nothing in isolation – each and every small change we make as individuals adds to the greater whole.

OUT ON THE LAND

❀ Hill Walking ❀ Keeping a Nature Journal
Foraging for Early Spring Greens and Herbs

This is an in-between time, a place on the edge. Winter is still with us, but within this is an awareness that spring will come soon. There are days of sheer magical brilliance when the skies are blue, the sun shines and calls us out onto the land. There are also dark days, of rain, fog, snow, ice and weather that lets us know we must wait a while longer before the transformation of spring fully begins.

This is the time when the ideas we have been incubating in the winter months, begin to rise in us. Like the life force of the land, everything is moving from the inside to the outside, from being held and cocooned in the dark, to an awakening into the light.

The Celtic festival of Imbolc celebrates 'First Stirrings' and the awakening of the life force. As you walk the land, look for where nature is stirring and also ask yourself what is stirring deep within you? What can you do now to set things in motion and help them to grow?

Walking helps the fluidity of the mind and beautiful places encourage our inspiration and muse. Carry a note book and pen with you on your walks so that you can write poetry and write down any inspiring thoughts that come to you, tapping into what is rising in you after your winter sleep.

Allow yourself to be pulled outside whenever the sun breaks through, delighting in the turn of the season. Get out for quick spins and feel the benefit of the quickening. Observe all that is stirring and see yourself part of the life force that is visibly on the move.

Hill Walking

Looking out across the landscape encourages our wider perspective and overview, so plan walks that take you high and give you long views. Once at the top, stay a while, sit and simply be in your surroundings. Let the vastness of the views expand your thinking and expand your sense of belonging to the vast interconnected web of life around you.

Keep a weather-eye always open and make sure you feel safe. This is where trusting your instincts and intuition is important. If you are inexperienced then take hill walking in stages. Begin with short trips at first and go out with someone experienced. Learn to map read so that at any given point you can get the map out and plan a route back.

Plan a vision quest for Imbolc. Look for what is stirring in you and take a long view of your life right now. What do you hope to achieve this year? What do you choose to put your energy into? Decide to do one thing to put this into motion.

Vision Quest, pages 15, 145

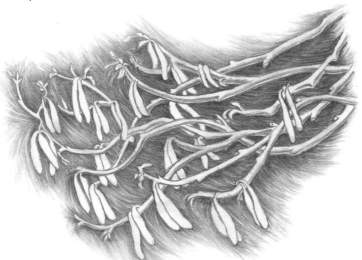

Keeping a Nature Journal

Keep a nature journal and write in the daily changes you observe around you. Keeping track of the weather is always interesting to look back on, as well as first sightings of birds and plants, first trees unfurling their leaves etc.

• Choose one tree to observe over a year. Document the year's cycle here, the seasonal changes in the environment and the wildlife. Document the bird and insect life, and the native plants growing near by. Write about the different atmospheres that different times of the year bring and how the tree changes in different weathers.

• Explore one place repeatedly, such as a spring, a cave, a lane. Make it your special place that you check in with and get to know intimately using all of your senses. Make a series of sketches or take photos from far away to close up. Observe its place in the environment, in the landscape, adding in any history that surrounds it. Let it feed your muse and write about it from your heart and feeling-self.

• Take photographs of the native plants, beginning now with the early spring plants. If you don't know their names then use the photos for identification and use a good field guide when you get home. This is the great advantage of digital photography. Label them on the computer and where you found them.

If you know their names then find out more about their herbal uses when you get home and whether they are edible.

Print off your best photos and add to your journal, along with the location and time of year. Add in anything you find out about the plant, so that your knowledge is always increasing. Add their locations to your local map.

Map Making, page 197

Foraging for Early Spring Greens and Herbs

Chickweed, Cleavers, Dandelion, Coltsfoot, Hairy Bittercress, Ribwort, Lady's Smock, Nettles, Sorrel, Wintercress, Wood Sorrel

As you walk keep an eye open for edible leaves to nibble along the way, or to gather and take home with you to add to the evening meal or to soup. Look out for herbs you can pick and dry for use as medicines, such as coltsfoot and ribwort, both good for coughs and chest complaints. Keep paper bags in your backpack for this purpose. Only pick from where there is a great profusion of plants and you feel confident it is wild and unsprayed.

Foraging, page 17
Drying Herbs, page 42

THE WILD GARDENER

❀ Early Edible Leaves ❀ Making a Wildlife Garden
❀ Making a Pond ❀ Native Pond Plants
❀ Container Gardening
❀ Guerrilla Gardening – Looking for Land

My daily maxim is "Sun's out, I'm out!" and this gets me outside in the garden for lots of short bursts of sunshine, activity and connection. It's good to see new plants surfacing and each time I go out there are more green leaves to add to my food.

Natural rainwater is so much better for plants than tap water. As well as connecting down pipes to water butts, leave out bowls and buckets and trugs to collect rain water. When they are full decant the water into plastic containers and water bottles.

This is the time of year for planning what you will give your attention to in the garden this coming year, planning what you want to grow, checking on the seeds you gathered in the autumn and ordering the seeds you need.

Early Edible Leaves

Corn Salad, Wintercress, Dandelion, Chickweed, Nettle, Sorrel and Wood Sorrel

During February more of the edible native plants can be found and picked in the garden if you grow them, or out on the land as you walk. They can also be covered by large plastic tubs or 5 litre (1 gallon) water bottles cut in half, to help bring them on quicker but don't forget to water them.

Dandelion leaves may be forced under large plant pots at this time of year. Cover the pot with straw or bubble wrap to encourage early young tender salad leaves.

Making a Wildlife Garden

Create a place in your garden that is dedicated to letting the wild edges of nature in. This needs to be a spot that can be left more or less to itself once created, perhaps towards the back of the garden. A wildlife area needs logs and stones for creatures to live under, and native plants left to go wild. Bird, insect and bee boxes can also be added.

Making a Pond

A pond is essential but if you have a very small garden a simple washing up bowl and some water mint is enough. Add a few rocks so that the birds can get a drink from it. Similarly if you decide to add some frogspawn, then make sure there is some way for the frogs to be able to get in and out when grown. The bowl can be sunk in the ground or stones and plants in pots placed around it will help disguise the bowl. It can also be painted green on the outside to disguise it further.

If you want a bigger pond then pond liners or thick pond plastic can be used. Think carefully where you want to put it before digging, as once in place it is not easy to move. If you put the pond in a dark corner, it tends to become murky from lack of light. We inherited the pond in our garden. It is right in the middle of the garden in a sunny spot. We walk past it every day and we often sit next to it. This means we are engaged with it and all its changing activity.

Once you have decided on location, shape and size, dig out the pond and line with at least 2cm (¾in) of fine sand, firmed down well, before laying in the liner. A shallow area means that the birds can bathe and the frogs can get in and out. Extra rocks can be added for this. Stones around the edges will anchor it and as soon as edge plants have become established, it will settle in and become part of the landscape of your garden.

If you know someone with a pond ask them for a few water snails – they will soon breed and will help to keep the pond clean. If you can find someone in the spring with frogspawn, these can be added and the frogs will live around your garden and return every year to lay more frogspawn. It is surprising how quickly pond insects arrive, including dragonflies to lay their eggs. The birds of course will be forever enjoying the water.

Native Pond Plants

Instead of imports from other countries buy native plants for the pond and pond edges.

Arrowhead (*Sagittaria sagittifolia*) – An attractive native perennial found in shallow water, canals and slow moving river edges. Pretty white flowers on spikes that grow up to 90cm (3ft) and leaves shaped like arrowheads.

Flowering Rush (*Butomus umbellatus*) – An attractive native perennial with white flowers, found in ponds, ditches, canals and river edges. Flowers July to September.

Frog-bit (*Hydrocharis morsus-ranae*) – An attractive native perennial of ponds and ditches with small white flowers that can also spread to pond edges.

Yellow Loosestrife (*Lysimachia vulgaris*) – An attractive native perennial of pond and river edges. Flowers July to August and grows to a height of approximately 1m (3ft 3in).

Yellow Flag Iris (*Iris pseudacorus*) – A native perennial of marshes and wet woodlands. A very attractive garden pond plant that will also grow in the soil around the edges.

Yellow Water Lily or Brandy Bottle (*Nuphar lutea*) – A native rhizome with beautiful yellow flowers that flower June to August.

Water Mint (*Mentha aquatica*) – A native perennial of marshes and ponds.

Water Violet (*Hottonia palustris*) – A native perennial found growing in ponds and ditches. It has beautiful pale lilac flowers that grow out of the water to a height of about 30-40cm (11-16in). Flowers May to June.

White Water Lily (*Nymphaea alba*) – A native rhizome with beautiful yellowy white flowers found in lakes, ponds and streams. The classic water lily with leaves floating on the top of the water.

Container Gardening

Plants can be grown in anything from old boots, crates, plastic tubs, old baskets, sacks, whatever you can lay our hands on and adapt. Old holdalls and large bags from charity shops are particularly good as the handles make them easy to move around. This is a good time to start gathering these and filling them up with soil and compost so that they are ready to start sowing seeds in when the weather warms up.

The Three Important Things to Remember Are...

1. Make drainage holes in the bottom, because plants hate their roots to be water logged.

2. Add other drainage materials in the bottom, stones, old broken crockery. Bark or shells make a lighter option if growing on a roof top.

3. Always use a good rich compost and feed regularly with a fertiliser, either home made or an organic seaweed fertilizer or organic chicken pellets.

Making Liquid Fertilisers, page 182

Guerrilla Gardening – Looking for Land

Scout out and about for land that could be used for guerrilla gardening this year. Look out for any neglected corners or verges, forgotten town planters, neglected traffic islands, land beneath high-rise flats or abandoned pockets of land that have become waste ground. There might be pieces of land that are 'grey areas', with no one particularly interested in them. Small, out of the way playgrounds can often do with a bit of beautification – talk to young mums and see if any are interested in growing herbs, flowers and some vegetables and making a garden along the edges.

Native plants have the power to break up concrete and make way for further planting. Throw some seed bombs filled with native plant seeds into the corners and along the edges of car parks, especially the more neglected ones and let nature do the rest. Look for places where nature has already begun to break up the concrete,. What other plants you could plant here later in the spring?

Making Seed Bombs, page 137

KITCHEN MEDICINE

❀ Spring Tonic Drink ❀ Coughs and Colds

❀ Elixirs and Tinctures

❀ Restoring Vital Energy

❀ Spring Green Pickle

❀ Winter Twigs

In the past when we live closer to nature, this would have been a lean time, the fruit and the roots that had been carefully stored beginning to run down and the preserves running low. But spring is just around the corner and already we are able to pick the first native spring greens.

Spring Tonic Drink

Both nettles and chives are growing now and both are rich in iron. Chickweed is high in vitamins A and C and high in iron, copper, magnesium and calcium. Pick the first nettle tops and chive shoots and a handful of chickweed and soak them in cold natural spring water overnight. This is a cold infusion. Drink the mineral and iron rich water as a spring tonic the next day and add the leaves to the soup pot. Top up the liquid to a pint and aim to drink 1 litre (2 pints) of natural spring water a day as a natural tonic and a spring clean for the whole system.

Spring Tonics, page 138

Coughs and Colds

This is the season of coughs and colds so drink the fruit syrups you made in the autumn to boost your vitamin C and check what dried herbs and tinctures you have that you can use. Elderberry tincture, syrup and elixir will help enormously. Hot elderberry wine before bed will help you to sweat and throw off a fever. Yarrow, elderflowers and mint is a classic combination for colds and flu. Vervain will help a cold to break and is great for convalescence.

Coughs can be treated with ribwort and coltsfoot, mullein, red clover, and rosehips. Honey's antibacterial quality rapidly clears infection and even when taken alone will help a cough or sore throat.

N.B. Do not give honey to babies under 12 months.

Making Your Own Cough Medicine, page 101
Cough Elixir, page 50

Elixirs and Tinctures

This is a good time to go through your tinctures and elixirs to check what you have made and used, and to check on their general condition. If any have sediment in the bottom of the bottle, carefully pour through double muslin or wine maker's filter paper, discard the bottom slurry, pour into a clean dark bottle and label.

If you find you are running short of something you can make it from dried herbs from your own store or bought from a herb suppliers. Soak them first in a little water to bring them back to life.

At this time of year there is time to play with herbal combinations depending on what you find you need. Combination elixirs can be made from tinctures by mixing them with equal amounts of honey and rebottling. It's a good way to use up the bits and bobs left over before the new season of available fresh herbs begins again. Check the list of herbs in 'Making Elixirs' to see what you might have that you can use.

Making Elixirs, page 48
Herb Suppliers, page 283

Restoring Vital Energy

It is easy to see how the cold and the damp seeps into our bones in the winter, creating stiff joints and dampening our sexuality. Lack of sunshine can bring depression and lack of energy. Keep a flame burning in your solar plexus, hara or belly. Remember to turn it on in the morning and picture yourself as a sensuous creative warm glowing person with a zest for life. Get in touch with what makes you feel beautiful and radiant and affirm you are lovable.

If the dark days are getting you down, then look in your store of dried herbs and tinctures to see what you might have to create a herbal restorative. The native plants St John's wort and vervain will add a lift to any mix, as well as mint, rose petals, nettle, cleavers and chickweed.

Create a refreshing pick-me-up by pouring boiling water on a fresh sprig of rosemary, chopped ginger, lemon and honey. This will stimulate the whole system, improve circulation and will send blood to the brain.

Don't forget to go outside frequently and take a daily walk, especially if the weather is wild! Seek out favourite places in your locality where you can revive, and take a long view and revel in being alive! Visit favourite trees you like to sit with, breathe deeply and look for signs of new life and the Earth awakening.

Spring Green Pickle

Chop up fresh dandelion leaves (taking out the bitter central stem), garlic mustard, chives and sorrel. Rinse them and without adding any water, steam gently for a minute to soften them. Then add cider vinegar and honey in equal measure. Chop in plenty of garlic, a little salt and ground black pepper. This makes a simple green pickle that can be added to any meal.

Winter Twigs

Bring a little of the outside in, cutting a few different coloured twigs and bring them in to the kitchen. In the warmth the buds will swell and leaves unfurl. Bring in some evergreens for the sheer delight of seeing their shiny green, their vigour and life force.

We are on the wild edge of spring and soon all life will be on the move, including yours. So savour this moment of gentle reflection, count your blessings and set new intentions for living closer to the Earth this coming year.

SEASONAL CELEBRATIONS

❀ Imbolc

❀ Making an Imbolc Doll or Earth Spirit

❀ Making a Set of Insight Stones

All around us are signs of the awakening Earth and the rising of the life force. Everything is moving from the inside to the outside, from being held and cocooned in the dark, to an awakening into the light. The ideas and longings we have been incubating during the winter months begin to rise in us, creating a bridge between our unconscious and what we consciously wish to bring into life.

Imbolc
End of January – Beginning of February

Imbolc is a festival to celebrate the light returning. It is also one of the great fire festivals of our ancient past and celebrates the rising of the creative life force and the spark of life from within.

The festival of Imbolc works directly with the energy of fire. Fire is the spark of life, the catalyst that sets things in motion and creates what happens next. It is the electric currents that course through the Earth and through every part of our bodies that stimulate us into action.

Fire inspires us to take risks, to be bold, to be spontaneous, to act on the strength of our convictions. We stand at a threshold of awakening potential and ask ourselves: what do we want from this new growth cycle?

At Imbolc we consciously fire up our new intentions, which propel us forwards and transform us from the inside. This is a great opportunity to change our relationship with the natural world, to see ourselves as part of nature and part of the web of life. We can choose to change our thinking patterns and our lifestyles, to begin to live with new values and create a new set of conditions from which to grow and change, so that we create a more harmonious and joyful future for ourselves and for the Earth.

Lay the foundation stones, set the corner post of how you want to live your life in the new cycle to come. Don't be complacent. Be adventurous. There is always more to change.

IMBOLC CELEBRATIONS

Included here are some ideas for connecting to the Earth, the seasonal energy, and your inner wisdom. Choose a couple of things to do, and be open to your own spontaneous inspirations of the moment.

For insights and overview about co-creating seasonal gatherings, see page 66

• Meet with friends for an Imbolc walk to see what is stirring in nature. Choose to go to a spring or site of a well or beautiful place that has a sacred feel. Reclaim your relationship with these places and send your love and thanks to the water flowing beneath the land. Take an offering or a special stone or crystal. Affirm that we are more than our surface reality, by speaking directly to the water, to the Earth and the Spirit of Place.

• After your walk, meet together around a fire, indoor or out and share homemade food. If you can't have a fire then fill a bowl with soil or sand and light plenty of candles.

• At the new moon invite friends round for an Imbolc evening. Invite everyone to bring food to share, a new candle and something that they have been doing, creating or making during the winter months. Each shares these things in the circle.

• Each light a candle for what brings you joy in your life. Start in a darkened room with just an Imbolc candle in a bowl of earth or compost at the centre of the circle. Gradually the room fills with light and people's joy.

• Each light a candle or two to celebrate the new ideas and the plans that are awakening in you at this time. Refine and stabilise these ideas and make new intentions to help set them in motion.

• Around the new moon, make time for reflection and meditation and to tune in to what is rising in you at this time. Be open to following your inspirations and the insights that rise from your intuitive self.

• Ask yourself what is your heart's true desire? What really inspires you? What do you long to do? Speak out about what you intend to do, " At this time of Imbolc I begin to ……… ", as you light a candle. Support the growth of these new seeds by daily appreciation of yourself and positive affirmations. Always visualise a positive outcome as if it has already happened. In this way you provide the best conditions for their future growth.

• Now is the time to be bold! Release your wild freedom and shed your old skin. What will block the flow of your new intentions? What conditioned patterns, excuses, old thought patterns limit you, and stop you moving forwards? Write them on pieces of paper and release them into the fire as you speak out loud and with determination: "I let go of………". Open up all possibilities and be open to growing in new ways this coming year.

• Each take a small stone and sit with it. Contemplate its great age and wisdom. While holding the stone ask what waits to be born? What longings do you carry within you? Name them in the circle and share your insights.

• Gather with your community and ask everyone to bring bottles of spring water to share. Spend some time tuning into the land from which they came. Each raise your glass to the Earth and the waters of the Earth and celebrate all that water means to you. Put a little of each of the spring waters in a central jug to share out at the end. Bless these waters and use for healing ceremonies in the future.

• Give thanks for being alive in these extraordinary times and pledge to be active in helping positive change to happen. Be prepared to step out in the service of the Earth, ready to do whatever we can do to make a difference, by speaking up and speaking out, speaking our truth through the words we choose, the decisions we make about where we put our energy and what we spend our money on.

• Share positive news you have heard about, so that more people become inspired and excited by positive change. Each person lights a candle for an aspect of the Earth that brings them joy and makes a solemn vow to be of service to this.

• Spend some time visioning the future you would like to live in. Vision the very best, the most wonderful, and the most heartwarming. Visualise the Earth healing and regenerating and a world wide movement for sustainability and care for our shared planet Earth. Anything is possible. As we vision these things they begin to have life. What will you do to support your vision?

Making An Imbolc Doll or Earth Spirit

Imbolc dolls are traditional at this time of year. They represent the new life that is growing in you and within the Earth. Push a large wooden bead or piece of elder onto a pointed stick to make the basic head and body of your doll and wrap fresh thin stems of willow, hazel, honeysuckle and ivy around this to create the arms and body shape. Use sheep's wool to wrap around the body to strengthen it, tie on some bits of material, leather, leaves, birch bark or raffia to make a skirt. Add moss, leaves or sheep's wool for hair.

Give your doll a seed sack to carry, made from a small circle of material in which you place your seeds of intention before tying it up. Write a message to yourself on a long thin piece of paper. Roll this up like a message scroll and tie it to your doll.

Making a Set of Insight Stones

Collect small flat stones or cut wooden rounds. Paint words on one side using acrylic paint. When the paint is dry, rub them with a very small amount of olive oil to bring out the colours and put them in a wide flat dish or in a pouch.

Every day or two, randomly pick a stone as you ask, "What do I need to nurture in myself today?" Allow the insight to guide and influence your actions through out the day. Encourage others to pick one too!

The words can also be written on cardboard leaves and kept in a pouch.

Insight words could include any of the following:

Trust; Peace; Simplicity; Love; Delight; Clarity; Understanding; Compassion; Community; Rest; Renewal; Intuition; Inspiration; Instinct; Loving Kindness; Transformation; Unity; Inner Wisdom; Truth; Joy; Vitality; co-operation; Hope; Happiness; Stillness; Acceptance; Non-judgement; Serenity; Healing; Spontaneity; Nourishment; Beauty; Protection; Courage; Strength; Regeneration; Fun; Relaxation; Appreciation; Co-creation; Sense of Wonder; Balance; Transition; Appreciation; Creativity; Playfulness; Flow.

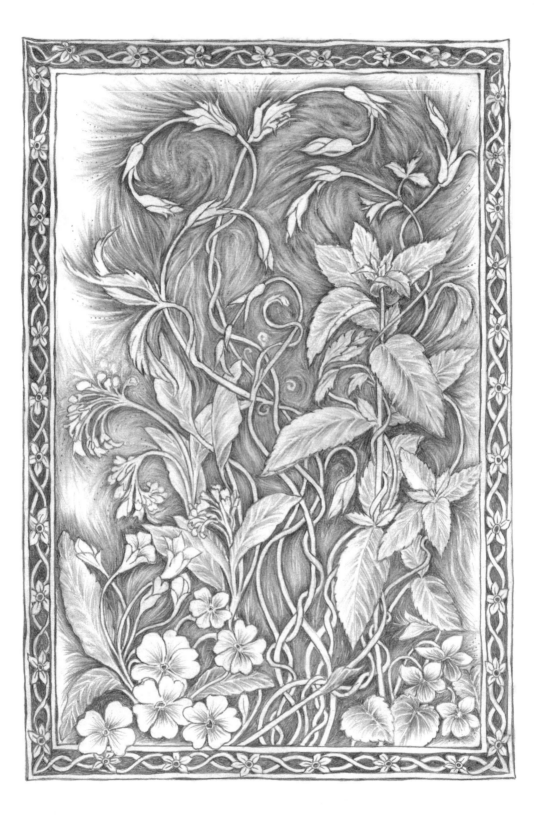

SPRING'S
wild edge

March into April

The Earth is changing fast now, responding to the increase in daylight. The sap is rising in the trees and they are getting ready for the great unfurling that is still to come. If we look closely we see that their buds are turning pink or purple and fattening up. Some briefly display their delicate flowers, which come before their leaves.

Spring in the air. There is a shift we can feel in our bones and taste on the breeze. It fills us with excitement and a need to get out and experience it. It can still be cold and unpredictable but we are also blessed with warm weather days that lift us up and expand our horizons. Wild weather days bring surprises. Winds blow away the winter debris, the rains refresh the land and new plants begin to grow, popping up almost over night.

Now is the time to begin! Boldness has genius! Begin this new cycle by stepping into your wilder edges. Leave behind old ways of thinking and see yourself as connected to the interconnected web of life. Look at everything you do, say, feel and think with fresh new eyes. Put changes in place every day by affirming the holistic perspective in every aspect of your life and lifestyle.

OUT ON THE LAND

❋ Hang Spring Cleaning! ❋ Night's Wild Edge
❋ Walking Alone ❋ Barefoot Walking
❋ Foraging for Medicinal Herbs and Edible Plants

Get up early for dawn walks that take you to high spots where you can watch the sunrise, now exactly in the East. This means getting out by about 5.30 in the morning, which is a great time to be out. The dawn chorus is a reward in itself, whether you see the sunrise or not, and it is a wonderful time to catch the early mists rising from the land and the bright green unfurling of leaves as nature awakes after its winter sleep.

The Spring Equinox is traditionally known as the first day of spring. Day and night become equal in both the Northern and Southern hemispheres. This point of balance in the Earth's yearly cycle holds many gifts for us to contemplate while out walking the land. It is an opportunity for us to look at how we can become more balanced and how we might live our lives with a greater awareness of our interconnectivity and our interdependency with the Earth. Aim to keep a balance between your heart and your mind.

Hang Spring Cleaning!

On bright spring days, down tools, abandon all jobs and set out for a walk, with a flask and a picnic packed in your day bag. Being outside is literally a breath of fresh air that re-energizes and feeds all of your senses. When the warm winds come, walk out onto moors and high land. Take in the long views and let the wind blow the cobwebs away. Climb high and feel your heart expand into the new spring season. You have to get out to do this, to fill your lungs with the fresh vital air of springtime. On bright cold days go walking in the woods. Find sheltered spots to sit in the sunshine with trees and lose yourself in nature and in the calm authority of the trees.

Contemplate the seeds you wish to sow in your own life as the time for new growth begins. Stay in touch with your inner longings. The interconnected life force can work in mysterious ways. Once your longing has life, then the potential for it to manifest is on the move. Ask yourself how you can begin to make this happen? Be open to flashes of inspiration and intuition beyond your logical mind. Let go of any limiting thoughts and be open to the power of miracles.

Night's Wild Edge

On fine dry evenings, and at the full moon, light a fire outside and invite friends to come and bring food and drinks to share. Wrap up warm, fire gaze, watch the stars, talk about what you know about them and our place in the solar system. These are always special evenings, times of deepening connection to ourselves, to the Earth and to each other.

Seize the moment and set off on 'night travels'. See if any friends will come with you. Agree to be quiet and not talk, so that you can hear the sounds of the night and the wildlife. Use hand signals to communicate and take a torch incase you need it.

Find your way from our over-lit night world to the places on the edge where the gentle natural light of the night can be found. In a town this may be harder but it can be done. Head for the river or canal and enjoy reflected light on the water. Head for the trees and the shadows they create. Explore the edges of what this brings up for you. Are your fears of walking at night grounded or are they a conditioned response? Open up the conversation and talk about it with friends.

Go a little further each time and gradually find your peace with the dark. Do it frequently, choosing darker nights when the moon isn't out until you become comfortable with this edge of your wild self.

Walking Alone

Decide to go walking alone. If you avoid doing this, perhaps you have a fear of it or have not yet discovered its delights. You may find that the self-imposed barrier is quickly dissolved. Being out alone means it is easier to become connected, both to yourself and the natural world around you. You can often be rewarded with glimpses of wildlife you would not have seen if you had been talking to a friend. You become more observant of nature, more spontaneous and go where you feel drawn.

Take a walking stick with you – it has so many uses while out walking. One that you have made yourself becomes like a companion and gives a little extra confidence to the lone walker.

Be open to the spirit of adventure and see where your feet take you! But also take an ordnance survey map with you and keep track of where you are from time to time, so that when you decide to, you can find your way back.

Find places to sit and watch the natural world go by. Develop the art of doing nothing, sit and observe and daydream.

Making a Walking Stick, page 215

Barefoot Walking

Walking barefoot makes you feel alive and becomes completely addictive! Choose an area of grassland that is easy on the feet. Early in the morning the cold is sharp and can even be briefly painful in a good way, but this soon disappears and is replaced by such a freshness and a delightful sense of connection and renewal.

Getting our feet in natural water, streams, springs and the sea, all bring the beneficial negative ions into our bodies. They are often very cold at this time of year but are so refreshing and reviving, it is well worth the experience.

Barefooting, page 130

Foraging for Medicinal Herbs and Edible Plants

Chickweed, Cleavers, Coltsfoot, Comfrey, Dandelion, Garlic Mustard, Hawthorn, Hop, Nettle, Ribwort, Ransoms, Sorrel

As you walk about, keep an eye open for herbs and plants to forage. The plants I list here are the ones covered by this book but of course there are many more.

Always carry brown paper bags in your pocket or bag because you never know what unexpected banks of native plants can be found when you are walking out and about at this time of year. Only pick plants where there are a lot of them, and make sure it is safe and acceptable to pick there. Otherwise decide to come back for a few seeds in the autumn and grow them at home next spring.

The woods are full of wild garlic, which can be added to any recipe and edible green mixtures. Eat what you have picked as part of your next meal or preserve them in vinegar, honey, alcohol, oil, or dry them for future use.

This is the best time for picking cleavers, a prime lymphatic tonic and cleanser that helps our bodies throw off toxins and pollutants. It is worth picking lots while they are at their best and drying them or making into tincture.

For medicinal uses of plants, see Plant Reference Guide, page 249

THE WILD GARDENER

❀ Edible Natives ❀ Sowing Seeds

❀ Growing Wild Flowers ❀ Tree Care

❀ Guerrilla Gardening – Seed Growing and Making Seed Bombs

I am out in the garden every day now, finding any excuse to be there. If the sun is out then I'm out! My maxim has carried me through the winter months and means my time outside is becoming even more frequent. Every excuse to be outside has to be acted on! Bunking off from boring indoor jobs is a priority! Catch up in the evening instead and give in to your deep instinct to be out in the fresh air. You have to be out there to experience the spring in its full glory.

The frogs have arrived in the pond, calling to each other day and night and creating copious amounts of frogspawn. Everywhere the birds are singing, nesting and claiming their territories. The dawn chorus is worth getting out of bed early to experience and listen out for the first chiffchaff, another herald of the arrival of spring.

Edible Natives

Cleavers, Chickweed, Corn Salad, Dandelion leaves, Dandelion flowers, Garlic Mustard, Hawthorn, Hairy Bittercress, Hop shoots, Ladies Smock, Primrose flowers, Sorrel, Salad Burnet, Violets, Wild Strawberry leaves, Wintercress, Wood Sorrel

The wild gardener is streaks ahead of her/his conventional cousins at this time of year. The so-called 'weeds' that begin to appear overnight are looked upon with glee, picked and eaten, and relished for their fresh spring energy. They can be used in salads long before we begin sowing our first cultivated lettuces and their flowers can also be eaten too. They are all at their best when eaten young at this time of year. They are the spring tonic herbs that help to clean out our systems and give us vital minerals we need to stay healthy. Try tasting them singularly first to learn their taste. Chop them up as part of a mixed leafed salad.

Weed them out as you make way for more conventional vegetables but always let one or two go to flower so they will reseed again.

Plant Reference Guide, page 249

Sowing Seeds

Sowing seeds begins in earnest now. Get out the seeds that you saved in the autumn, remembering what you know about the plants, their preferred habitat and uses. Revisit your herbal notebooks and last year's gardening notebooks. Check in with other gardening friends what seeds they might have to spare before you order more seeds. Organise an impromptu seed-swop supper!

Sow seeds of edible salad plants in any wild and wacky container you can find, from old holdalls to old boots. Make drainage holes in the bottom and fill with good compost. Plan to create a feast outside your door! Be aware that if you buy plug plants they may have been sprayed. Check if you buy non-organic seeds, that they have not been coated with neonicatinoids that harm the bees and other insects.

Set up a potting table in the sunshine where you have seed trays, clean pots and compost ready. If you have a greenhouse you are lucky; without one you have to be more inventive. Impromptu cloches can be made out of large plastic storage boxes turned upside down. They act as mini green-houses for protecting seeds in seed-trays or pots of seedlings and are ideal for keeping on the patio or outside your door where you can keep an eye on them. Put a thick layer of cardboard on the ground beneath the trays and check them regularly for any slugs sleeping under them. Lift the tubs up in hot weather to let the air circulate and remember to keep your seedlings regularly watered. Once danger of frost is over, the plants can be put on top of the tubs to harden them off for planting, and out of the reach of slugs. In the summer these tubs are ideal for use as temporary water containers to store rain water.

Remember to give thanks as you plant your seeds. Fill yourself up with your appreciation and love for them, for their medicine and for feeding you. Plant your visions, hopes and seed-ideas as you plant your seeds. Plant extra seeds to give to friends and family. Plant seeds with children. Teach them about growing food and growing flowers.

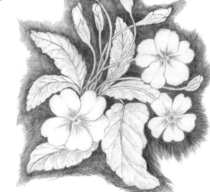

Growing Wild Flowers

This year grow some native wild flower seeds and create a cottage garden – even in a pot. These plants once grew everywhere and by growing them you will help the bees and butterflies to thrive. Many of these plants have now become rare in the wild so if you have plants to spare plant them out in any edge-place, their seeds will help to re-establish them in our countryside. There are no guarantees that these will take outside of their native habitats, but plants are adaptable and your success could save a dwindling species. Look up the kind of habitats they prefer in the wild and anything that can help you to grow them successfully. Once you have established them and have seed to share then let people know what you have. Seeds are easy to put in the post!

The following plants are all native wild flowers that will look good growing in any garden or could be grown for reintroducing back into the wild.

N.B. These are not listed for their edible and medicinal uses. Use a good foraging guide and herbal to find out more about them. Some are covered in the Plant Reference Guide, page 249.

Some Native Annuals

Cornflower or Bluebottle (*Centaurea cyanus*) – Lovely garden plant that flowers June to August.

Corn Chamomile (*Anthemis arvensis*) – Grows in fields and likes an open position. Flowers June to July.

Field Poppy (*Papaver rhoeas*) – Grows in disturbed ground. Flowers May to August.

Common Forget-me-not (*Myosotis arvensis*) – An all time favourite that will grow anywhere. Flowers April to September.

Wild Candytuft (*Iberis amara*) – Grows on dry hillsides and grasslands. Flowers July to August.

Wild Pansy or Heartsease (*Viola tricolor*) – Sometimes a perennial, prefers sandy soils. Flowers April to September.

Yellow Rattle (*Rhinanthus minor*) – Grows in grasslands and waysides. Flowers May to August.

Some Native Perennials

Agrimony (*Agrimonia eupatoria*) – Found in hedgebanks and roadsides. Flowers June to August.

Betony (*Stachys officinalis*) – Found in woods and hedgerows. Flowers June to September.

Bistort or Easter-ledges (*Polygonum bistoria*) – Grows along roadsides and in meadows. Previously eaten at Easter with hard boiled eggs. Flowers May to August.

Cowslip (*Primula veris*) – Found in meadows and hedgebanks. Flowers April to May.

Common Mallow (*Malva sylvestris*) – Found in wasteland and hedgerows. Flowers June to September.

Marsh Mallow (*Althaea officinalis*) – Found in salt marshes and ditches near the sea, but will grow outside of these conditions. Flowers July to September.

Columbine (*Aquilegia vulgaris*) – Found in woods and damp places but now rare in the wild. Flowers May to June.

Field Scabious or Gypsy Rose (*Knautia arvensis*) – Found growing in dry grasslands and roadsides. Flowers June to September.

Harebell or Scottish Bluebell (*Campanula rotundifolia*) – Found growing in dry grassy places, hedgebanks and roadsides. Flowers July to September.

Jacobs Ladder (*Polemonium caeruleum*) – Flowers May to June.

Maiden Pink (*Dianthus deltoides*) – Flowers June to September.

Meadow Cranesbill (*Geranium pratense*) – Found along roadsides and in hedgebanks. Flowers May to September.

Meadowsweet (*Filipendula ulmaria*) – Found in wet meadows, marshes and along riversides. Flowers June to August.

Nettle-leaved Bellflower or Throatwort (*Campanula trachelium*) – Flowers June to September.

Ox Eye Daisy, Dog Daisy or Marguerite (*Leucanthemum vulgare*) – Found growing in grasslands and along roadsides. Flowers May to August.

Primrose (*Primula vulgaris*) – Found in woods and on hedgebanks. Flowers March to May.

Purple Loosestrife (*Lythrum salicaria*) – Found growing along damp watersides. Flowers June to August.

Salad Burnet (*Sanguisorba minor*) – Found in grasslands and meadows. Flowers May to August.

Self Heal (*Prunella vulgaris*) – Found growing in grass, along roadsides and in woodland clearings. Flowers June to September.

Sneezewort (*Achillea ptarmica*) – Found in damp meadows and roadsides. Flowers July to August.

Stonecrop, English (*Sedum anglicum*) – Found on rocks, in walls, shingle, dunes and dry grassland. Flowers June to July.

St Johns Wort (*Hypericum perforatum*) – Found in hedgerows, woodlands and along grassy banks. Flowers June to September.

Sweet Violet (*Viola odorata*) – Found along wood edges and in hedgebanks. Flowers February to April.

Sweet Woodruff (*Galium odoratum*) – Found in woods and shady edges. Pretty banks of flowers from April to June.

Toadflax (*Linaria vulgaris*) – Found in wasteland, roadsides, hedgerows and grasslands and also grown in gardens. Flowers June to September.

SOME NATIVE BIENNIALS

These take 2 years to come to maturity and don't flower in the first year. Once established though, there are plants flowering every year.

Foxglove (*Digitalis purpurea*) – Found in woods, hedgerows and open places. Flowers June to September.

Mullein or Aaron's Rod (*Verbascum thapsus*) – Also known as Aaron's Rod – found on sunny banks and waste places. Flowers June to August.

Viper's Bugloss (*Echium vulgare*) – Found on dry soils, grassy places, sea cliffs and dunes, waste places. Flowers June to September.

Weld (*Reseda luteola*) – Found along roadsides, wasteland, fields and is an ancient bright yellow dye plant. Flowers June to August.

Native Plant, Seed and Bulb Suppliers, page 283
For edible and medicinal uses, see Plant Reference Guide, page 249

Tree Care

The sap is beginning to rise in the trees now and it is too late now to cut them hard back or dig them up to move them. This will have to wait now until the winter.

The trees in pots that have been wintering in the sunny spots can now be moved as you need these spots for seed growing. As the weather improves, and once danger of frost has gone, put bowls under them and remember to water them in dry weather.

If you have planted native trees out this winter, you must follow this up with caring for them throughout their first year while their roots become established. Keep the grass clear around their base and water in dry weather.

Guerrilla Gardening – Seed Growing and Making Seed Bombs

Growing native plant seeds to reintroduce back into the wild is an aspect of guerrilla gardening I love. This will help the bees, especially if you choose the wild flowers they love to visit. Choose to buy some seeds from the list above or use the seeds you collected in the autumn.

SEED GROWING

Sprinkle seeds into homemade cardboard tubes or loo rolls filled with a good quality compost. Put each one in a small sandwich bag and stack them side by side in plastic food trays. Giving them their own bag makes it easier for planting out as the cardboard roll disintegrates. This creates seed-cluster plugs, which are easy to transport for planting out. Slice into the ground with a sharp thin bulb-planting trowel and slot in the seed-cluster, cardboard roll and all (but not the plastic bag obviously).

MAKING SEED BOMBS

Using a mixture of sand, clay and compost, mix with native wild flower seeds and then add a little water and press them into balls. Leave to harden off a little in egg boxes, but it is good if they are still damp inside. It is always best to scatter them when it's likely to rain. The seed bombs can be thrown along field edges, and any other place you can find in your locality where there is already some soil and native flowers have a chance of growing. The success rate isn't high but they are such fun!

Don't forget the aftercare, going out with watering can or bottle of water to give the plants a drink if it is dry and in some cases weeding around them while they become established. Choose places to plant that you walk by often so that you can keep an eye on how they are doing.

Choose to grow native plants that are hardy and fit the places you are planting them out in.

KITCHEN MEDICINE

❀ The Spring Tonic Herbs ❀ Making Leaf Tinctures

❀ Herbal Elixirs – Iron tonic, Digestive tonic

❀ Flower Essences ❀ Infused Leaf Oils

❀ Edible Greens – Green Pies ❀ Green Smoothie

❀ Nettles – Nettle soup – Green Pesto

❀ Garlic Mustard – Green Dips and Mayonnaise

❀ Spring Clean, Clutter Clear and Simplify ❀ Spring Posies

There are so many medicinal and edible plants growing now and it is so good to be using the fresh plants again. Now is the time to start eating up all those jams, chutneys and stored preserves you made last year. Once you have fresh things growing it is easy to forget your store cupboard and then things can go to waste. There is something very satisfying about seeing the shelves of stored preserves become bare again, knowing that a new cycle is about to begin.

The Spring Tonic Herbs

Dandelion, Chickweed, Chives, Cleavers, Nettle

These spring tonic herbs are thriving now. They cleanse the blood, strengthen the liver and gently detox the body after the heavier foods of winter. Eat them every day from now until they become too tough in early summer. Chop them up and make sweet green salads with a little honey, some garlic and balsamic vinegar. Add them to soups, scatter over standard salads, and chop finely as a green garnish. Some of them can be quite fiery or bitter so mix them with dressings and chutneys or chop fine and sprinkle over other food. They are a great gift from nature and not to be wasted!

The secret of growing and eating native plants is to be inventive. Substitute some natives instead of conventional salad leaves and invent new ways to eat them that you really like. So many of them are kidney and liver tonics that will help our bodies throw off toxins and modern day pollutants, so it is worth putting some into your food every day. They can also be dried for herb teas and for adding to food in the winter months.

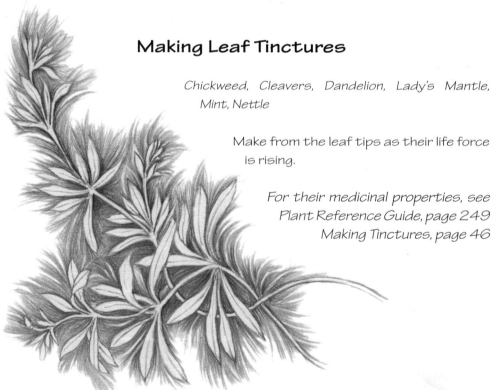

Making Leaf Tinctures

Chickweed, Cleavers, Dandelion, Lady's Mantle, Mint, Nettle

From the leaf tips as their life force is rising.

For their medicinal properties, see Plant Reference Guide, page 249 Making Tinctures, page 46

Herbal Elixirs

Chickweed, Cleavers, Dandelion, Lady's Mantle, Mint, Nettle

Any of the above plants can be made into elixirs. Add something aromatic that supports the overall properties of the herbs.

IRON TONIC ELIXIR

Nettles, Chives, Chickweed and Lady's Smock

The main herbs that are strong in iron are available now and it is worth making this valuable iron tonic from the fresh herbs.

DIGESTIVE TONIC ELIXIR

Mint, Chickweed, Dandelion, Hops, Red Clover, Vervain, Thyme, Rosemary, Lavender, Lemon Balm, Fennel

Use any of these fresh leaves for this invaluable digestive tonic.

Making Honey Elixirs, page 48

Flower Essences

Making flower essences is a simple way to connect to the beauty and essential energy of a plant. They can be used to support the actions of the herbs and can also be made from any flower you are attracted to including those that are not safe to ingest. Intuit for yourself their message to you and enjoy admiring and connecting to the plant and sitting in the sunshine as the remedy infuses.

Making a Flower Essence, page 38
For Metaphysical Uses, see Plant Reference Guide, page 249

Infused Leaf Oils

Chickweed, Chives, Cleavers, Comfrey

Herbal oils are simple to make and the herbal properties of the plants are absorbed through the skin. Only make small amounts that you know you will use.

Making Herbal Oils (Macerations), page 53

CHICKWEED OIL

Its action is cooling and soothing. Use to cleanse and to draw out poisons from any inflamed skin conditions and for burns.

CHIVE OIL

Rich in iron and a great antiseptic. This oil can also be used in salad dressings.

CLEAVERS OIL

Benefits dry skin, psoriasis and dandruff and good for any sores and blisters. Boosts the immune system.

COMFREY OIL

Use for all swellings, sprains, torn ligaments and to mend broken bones (once they have been set by a professional). This herb will heal in record time so be sure the wound is clean.

Edible Greens

Cleavers, Chickweed, Chives, Corn Salad, Dandelion, Garlic Mustard, Hawthorn, Hairy Bittercress, Hop shoots, Ladies Smock, Nettle tops, Sorrel, Salad Burnet, Wintercress

As I weed out the native plants to make way for my conventional vegetables to grow, I save the edible leaves to make a spinach-type mixture at the end of a day's gardening, adding conventional spinach leaves too. If I go for a walk I forage for edible greens and add these in too. This cooked mixture can be added to risottos, stir-fries and for making 'Green Pie'.

GREEN SPINACH-TYPE MIXTURES

1. Gather a colander of mixed edible greens from the garden or safe location. Include garden spinach if you have it. Wash and carefully sort through the leaves, discarding any that don't look right, are diseased or have eggs or insects living on the back of them. Return these to the earth.

2. Put the wet leaves in a pan and gently steam them for a few minutes with the lid on, turning frequently with a fork.

3. When all the leaves have softened, strain off the liquid and press the greens with the back of a wooden spoon to squeeze out more liquid. Save the bright

green liquid to add to sauces or for stock.

4. The cooked spinach-mix will keep in a tub the fridge for 3-5 days. Label and date it if you are busy in the garden every day! Or it can be frozen if you have a freezer.

Green Pie

1. Prepare the spinach-type mixture as above.

2. Chop the cooked greens with a knife and fork.

3. Place the chopped greens in a bowl and add a couple of beaten eggs, some grated strong cheddar, (also good with a blue cheese), and some finely chopped onions and garlic. Mix it all together and add seasoning.

4. Line a pie dish with pastry, pour in the mixture and bake in a medium oven for 25 minutes until the mixture has set.

Green Feta Pie

1. Alternatively crumble goats cheese into the cooked spinach-type mixture and add one egg. Season with lots of coarse sea salt, black pepper and Cajun spice.

2. Pile into a pastry base and add a pastry lid. Sprinkle with sea salt and sprigs of thyme.

3. Bake for 25 minutes.

Serve either of these pies hot with new potatoes and salad, or equally good cold for lunch the next day or a slice as a snack.

Green Smoothie

This is a great way to take your spring tonic herbs! Liquidise a mix of plant leaves, milk and some yogurt. I add chopped garlic too. It packs a punch and gives your whole immune system a boost. Or add a couple of teaspoons of honey also good for the immune system and extra immune system tinctures such as cleavers, elderberry, nettles, self heal, rosehip and borage.

Nettles

Nettles are growing fast now so make good use of the iron and mineral-rich nettle tops. They can be added to any cooked spinach mixes or made into nettle dishes in their own right. They can be picked and made into tincture or dried for future nettle teas.

Making Tinctures, page 46
Drying Herbs, page 42
Nettles, page 268

NETTLE SOUP
Everyone has their own favourite version of nettle soup. Traditionally potatoes are used, but this recipe uses chick peas instead.

1. Pick, wash and drain nettle tops.

2. Sweat an onion or two, or any leeks that need eating before they bolt.

3. Add the nettle tops and water, a generous amount of stock powder or cube, and cook for ten minutes.

4. When cooked, add a drained tin of chick peas (or potatoes), lots of finely chopped garlic, soya sauce and black pepper.

5. Liquidise, or mash with potato masher.

6. Always improved by a generous swirl of cream or soya cream and sprinkled with black pepper before serving.

The above recipe can be used for any green soup, incorporating any edible greens.

NETTLE AND CHICKWEED PESTO
Pick a quantity of nettle and chickweed tops. Put in a blender with a handful of pine nuts or ground nuts of your choice, two cloves of chopped garlic and olive oil to make a paste. Parmesan can also be added. Any other green herb can be added.

Green Pesto
Add in any other edible greens such as cleavers, chickweed, sorrel, salad burnet.

Nettle Risotto
Make in the usual way adding chopped nettles near the end to keep their lovely colour.

Garlic Mustard or Jack by the Hedge

This plant gives a good garlic flavouring for sauces. The leaves can be eaten raw in salads or placed directly in cheese sandwiches but it is very hot. They can also be added to spinach type mixes, stews and soups.

GARLIC MUSTARD DIP

115g (4oz) of curd cheese, or any soft cheese, or sour cream
4 tablespoons of fresh chopped garlic mustard
2 tablespoons of chopped chives

Beat the cheese and chopped herbs in a bowl and add salt and black pepper to taste.

GREEN DIPS

Use chickweed, cleavers, lady's smock, salad burnet, sorrel, chives, and make in the same way.

GARLIC MUSTARD MAYONNAISE

1 egg yolk
½ teaspoon Dijon mustard
2 tablespoons fresh chopped garlic mustard
125ml (4 fl oz) of olive oil
1 tablespoon white wine vinegar

Method
1. Chop the garlic mustard.

2. Whisk the egg yolk, mustard and garlic mustard.

3. Gradually add the oil and vinegar in small amounts.

4. Add more vinegar, salt and pepper to taste.

Green Mayonnaise

Use chickweed, chives, cleavers, lady's smock, salad burnet, sorrel, garlic, winter cress, and make in the same way.

Simplify, Spring Clean and Clutter Clear

Traditionally this is the time for a spring clean of your living space, to throw open the windows and let in the fresh air, to release what may be stuck or stagnant, and prepare for the new season ahead. It is a good time to cast off emotional baggage too and let the spring winds carry away the old parts of yourself that you no longer wish to encourage.

Look for how you can simplify your life, your home, your expectations of yourself and others expectations of you. Many of us have too many possessions, so have the pleasure of giving things away to friends when you know they would like something that you no longer use. Your generosity will encourage others to be generous too.

Spring Posies

Pick small posies of the first spring flowers and bring them into the kitchen, where you frequently stand to cook or on the kitchen table. On dark inside days they serve to gladden your heart and remind you that spring is here.

SEASONAL CELEBRATIONS

✤ Spring Equinox

✤ Making a Nest ✤ Making a Bead Necklace

As the new growth cycle begins, use this prime time to begin new projects and to sow the seeds of the future you wish to see happen. This is a prime time to put things into motion that we want to manifest this year.

By your every action, by the thoughts you encourage and the words you say, you make fertile all the things you have carried with you in your heart throughout the winter. Begin to put plans into action and sow new seeds of yourself, your future, and the future of the Earth. As we sow our new seeds we must also consider what they need in order to grow, give them the right conditions for healthy growth and let go of the things that we know will hamper their growth.

Spring Equinox
21st – 23rd March

The Spring Equinox is a celebration of spring, new life, fertility and birth. Originally a celebration of the goddess Eostara, and the fertility of women, the egg is her symbol, which represents all that we bring into life.

At the Equinox, day and night are equal in length, reminding us of the need to balance our inner and outer selves, our receptive and active selves, our intuition and our logic and find ways to firmly establish this balance in our lives.

Spring Equinox is a celebration of the fertility that comes from the union of opposites: dark and light, sun and rain, warmth and cold, inner and outer, receptive and active, male and female. From our conscious blending of these separate parts of ourselves, a new holistic perspective will grow.

SPRING EQUINOX CELEBRATIONS
Included here are some ideas for connecting to the Earth, the seasonal energy, and your inner wisdom at this time. Choose a couple of things to do, and be open to your own spontaneous inspirations of the moment.

For insights and overview about co-creating seasonal gatherings, see page 66

•   Gather with friends for a Spring Equinox celebration. Arrange to meet and walk to a high spot to experience the Equinox dawn together, now directly in the East.

Name what you bring into balance in your life. Bring breakfast food and drinks to share, out on the land if it is fine, or back at someone's house if not.

•   On the Equinox, or as near as you can make it, put aside a whole day to walk in nature, with friends or alone, depending on your need. Your walk may take the form of a pilgrimage, Vision Quest or Wonder Wander. Plan it ahead so that you know you will go out on this day. Be open to whatever the day brings and aim to go whatever the weather. Set off early with simple food and drink, a notebook, a compass, a walker's map. Walk with mindful spontaneity and have an Equinox adventure!

Pilgrimage, Vision Quest, Wonder Wander, page 15

• Spend some time reflecting on the new seeds you wish to grow in your life right now. What new projects would you like to start? Be bold and shine! Name these: "At this time of Spring Equinox I plant the seed of........."

Plant these new seeds of intention with a vision of them complete and whole. Know that they will manifest. Doubt, and fear will inhibit their growth. Trust and certainty will give them energy.

• The inner seeds you plant also need watering, nurturing, tending and attention to help them to grow. Ask yourself what do these seeds need to grow? What will prevent them from growing? Name the old parts of yourself that you leave behind, that you will no longer give any energy to. Then name what new parts of yourself you will encourage to grow.

• Invite friends for an Equinox gathering. Ask everyone to bring food and drink to share. This may be out on the land, in the garden or indoors depending on the weather. Make a central focus of spring flowers and candles.

• Reflect on what you need to bring into balance in your life right now. Write about this in your journal and share the central core of your understanding with each other.

• Whatever you give your energy to right now will grow. Ask yourself how you can make simple and joyful lifestyle changes that will not only improve the quality of your life, but will help to heal the planetary imbalances of our time. Write about this in your journal and share the key points with each other.

• Everything we do makes a difference, as all things are connected, and once you change one thing, there is no knowing where or who this will influence, and help create more change. Begin simply by choosing a few things you could change easily. Share these with each other.

• Gather in a circle and pass round a basket of small Fairtrade chocolate eggs.

Each take one and name the egg of potential that you will nurture in your life and in the world. The basket can go round several times if there are enough eggs.

• Celebrate each other's plans, encourage, offer help and support each other to begin.

• Pass round a basket of coloured ribbons. Each take a ribbon for each thing you wish to change in yourself or about your lifestyle that will help the Earth. Hang them in a tree in your garden or nearby.

• Pass round a basket of seeds, which people can take away with them to plant. As you take a seed, name what you intend to do to help the Earth. The large seeds work best, such as: sunflowers, nasturtiums, peas, mangetout or any bean.

• Ask everyone to bring compost, plant pots and native seeds to the gathering. Each choose to grow a different native plant. Sprinkle a few seeds in each pot and write on the pot with a white-out pen or decorate them with acrylics. Find out as much as you can about the plant you grow, sharing this with the group when you meet next. Share the plants with the group when they have become established.

• Meet in the evening and aim to have a fire if it is fine. Ask everyone to bring seasonal food and pots of native plants to share. Plan future guerrilla gardening activities and share what each knows about the plants and why you bought them. Set out on an evening of guerrilla gardening and plant out your plants.

Making a Nest

A small nest can be made to hold your Equinox eggs and wishes.

Using willow, dogwood or any other lengths of flexible material, weave three circles, each a little smaller than the next.

Using thread or raffia, tie these together to make a small nest.

Place the nest on a piece of birch bark or put pieces of birch bark inside to stop everything falling out, and add twigs, grasses, and finally a little bit of moss to make a cushion for your eggs.

Have a bowl of small chocolate eggs ready and as each person takes an egg they say out loud what they are nurturing within them and what their new intentions are, and places the egg in their nests.

Making a Bead Necklace

1. Gather some twigs from Native trees, spending time with the trees first and asking for a gift of wood from each tree. Intuit what each tree means to you and be open to its message-gift. You might find fresh windblown wood beneath the tree. If it has its leaves still attached then it is perfect for making beads.

For more about the significance of different native tree woods, see Making a Talking Stick, page 240

2. Saw into small bead lengths. Gently poke a hole through each bead with a bradawl or drill holes with a small drill bit.

3. Spend time working the beads with a penknife and sandpaper, taking off the bark or some of the bark, and sanding the wood with three grades of sandpaper – starting with rough sandpaper to smooth out the penknife marks, then moving on to medium to begin the smoothing process, and finishing with fine to bring the wood to a really fine smooth finish.

4. To bring out the colour of the wood and feed and protect it, finish off by oiling your beads. I use any of the infused herbal oils I have made. This brings another layer of energy to the beads.

St John's Wort Oil – For protection and supporting transitions.

Chickweed Oil – For creating connection, increased receptivity and compassion.

Dandelion Oil – For clearing emotional stagnation and increasing adaptability.

Elder Leaf Oil – For throwing off old stuck energy, to move fears and bring clarity.

Rose Petal Oil – For love.

5. Use a strong thread, fine leather, or fine elastic and thread on the beads to make a necklace or bracelet. As you thread each bead on, bring the qualities of the wood into your heart to help you in your quest to become part of the Earth's human support system. Bring in your growing awareness of the interconnected web of life. As we each begin to make this shift, we give birth to positive change in the world.

6. Alternatively, gather lots of beads made from natural materials, such as semi precious stones and crystals, wood, shell, glass, metal. If you do this with others, ask everyone to bring beads to share. Agree to stay in focused silence, perhaps with music playing that helps you deepen and expand inwards. As you thread, choose each bead to represent each of the blessings you have in your life and your appreciation for the many aspects of the Earth you love and value.

7. When you are finished, write in your journal what your necklace means to you and what was revealed as you made it. If you are with friends, when everyone has finished, have a go-round and share this with each other. Have a simple ceremony to dedicate your necklace.

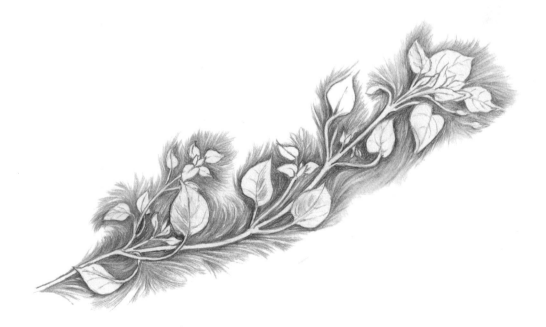

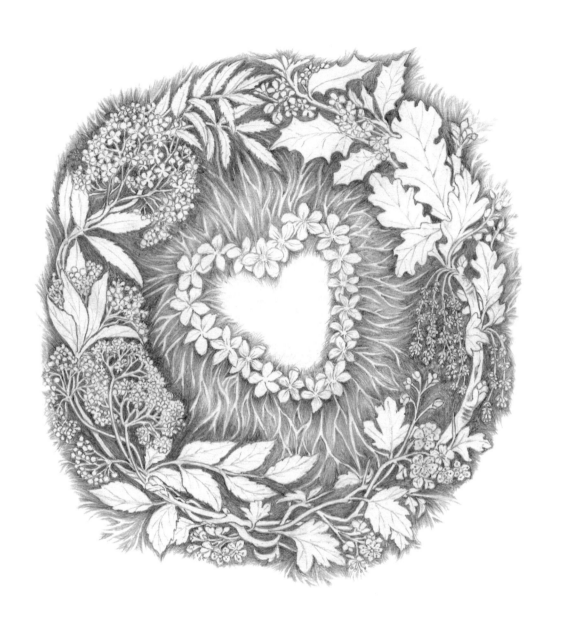

on the edge of
SUMMER

April into May

This is the beginning of summer, the great fertile time, when the interconnected web of life is at its most visible and accessible. The trees come into leaf and the land becomes green again. Life is on the move, wild and untamed, mysteriously profound in its ability to simply let go and grow. We are called to get out from the confines of buildings and engage with the life force, become part of its power to go wild, grow and manifest.

Allow for the unexpected and the spontaneous! Jump in and experience life at its most sensuous, alive and fertile. Push the boundaries of each of your senses so that you live each day with the recognition that there is so much more to experience, there on the margins of our previously perceived known world and understanding.

Manifestation is at its height so look at what you are manifesting in your life through the words you say, the thoughts you repeat to yourself and the beliefs you hold. Whatever we give our attention to will grow. Walk towards all things that will support your highest good and the highest good of the Earth. Be clear of your intentions and what you choose to give your power, energy and time to.

It is a wildly busy time, so take time out to walk the land, slow down and contemplate these things, while remaining open to all the abundance and subtleties of the life force manifesting around you.

OUT ON THE LAND

❀ The Art of Seeing ❀ Finding Springs and Wells

❀ Making Flower Essences from the Native Trees

❀ Foraging for Edible Greens and Medicinal Herbs

All of life is expanding, moved by the increase in daylight and the heat of our sun, now entering its final phase of its year's cycle. This is a period of rampant growth energy, when the sheer abundance and beauty of the natural world is overwhelming and deeply moving in its robustness and fragility. It marks the transition between the end of spring and the beginning of summer.

The Celtic festival of Beltain is a celebration of the life force and the abundant fertility of the Earth. Traditionally it was known as a time when we can slip between the worlds and meet with elementals and nature spirits. It is as if life cannot contain the normal boundaries in this rapid expansion of growth and the wild edges of our expected reality become blurred.

The Art of Seeing

Drawing and painting out in nature is very much about the art of 'seeing' and of 'being', enjoying the flow of the moment, entering into interrelationship and communion with the natural world.

We can all draw or paint, we just have to drop the critical voice inside us, laid down so long ago and remind ourselves that drawing and painting is not about the destination, the finished picture – it is about the journey. In fact an unfinished picture is often more satisfying and pleasing to the eye.

Instead of being frustrated by your lack of skill at catching a true likeness, choose to catch the flavour, catch the feeling that a place gives you, the patterns you see. Create your own style that you enjoy doing and enjoy looking at. If something is not looking how you want it to, then turn the page and start again. Old unfinished pictures can be added to at another time. Don't show your work to other people unless you want to. Do it for you and you alone. The more you do, the more confident you will grow.

The first thing is to find a good place to sit. Begin by doing nothing other than looking. Simply slow down and absorb the benefits of being outside and feeling yourself to be part of nature and not separate from it. Maybe you need to be with the long view or to look at the plants and trees close to. Creative flow will emerge from what inspires you in the moment.

Drawing or painting gives a place or a tree or a plant your full attention. All life responds in a positive way to positive input. Sometimes things can happen in these in-between times – a deep connection and understanding with the natural world is experienced, a sense of communion with a plant, tree or place, or an insight gained.

Finding Springs and Wells

Springs are a wild edge between earth and water. The water may have travelled for hundreds of miles in underground channels, for hundred of years, filtered and energised by the Earth before it comes to the surface in this moment.

Visiting the sites of old springs and wells gives us a chance to give our thanks to water. In the past they were honoured, dressed with flowers and traditionally visited at Beltain. Many are still there and forgotten. Check old town maps to see where they might have been in the town and see if there is any evidence of their survival. This can take you on an adventure of discovery and reconnection.

Make a pilgrimage to visit any that are still in use, where you can take bottles and collect the water. Many springs and wells were reputed to have healing powers, and are rich in minerals and trace elements coming from deep within the Earth. Many can still be found alongside churches or are still there on the edges of villages and sites of ancient communities. Other springs can be found by looking on old ordnance survey maps.

Young streams can be followed back up into the hills to find their source spring. Follow the sound of the water, keeping it in your consciousness and letting it lead you and absorb you. Listen to its many voices and observe its flowing patterns. Once you find the place where the water comes out of the ground, find somewhere to rest and to breathe in the special and beneficial negative ions and minerals rising fresh from within the Earth. Get your shoes and socks off and get them in the water. Meditate a while and see what comes to you here in this special edge place. Be open to your intuitive responses. Become aware of its 'Genius Loci', its 'Spirit of Place' and be open to your connection to this.

If this is a pilgrimage or Vision Quest, or part of your Beltain celebration, take a gift, such as a stone or crystal, something made from clay or wood. This is an age-old tradition. Sit a while and absorb and observe everything around you. Ask for inspiration for your new journey and see what comes to you. The negative ions that moving water and light create are also beneficial to us, so just being there helps us to heal and regenerate.

Take three ribbons with you to hang in a nearby hawthorn tree to give thanks for the water, for the Earth and for your life, affirming new intentions and healing.

Libations and Offerings, page 199

Making Flower Essences from the Native Trees

There is something so touching about the native trees in flower. They are often delicate and unassuming for such large beings and they are often short-lived and can be missed.

You will need a small glass bowl, a small jug, a small bottle of spring water, and a dark dropper bottle that is half filled with brandy. Place the small glass bowl filled with spring water beneath the tree in a sunny spot or up in a crook of a branch where it will catch the sun light. Sit near the tree and appreciate its beauty. See what comes to you as you allow its vital presence to filter through you. Often this will release understanding about the tree's essential energy and a realization of what you might need in your life right now.

Thank the tree before leaving. The essence can be taken daily to help anchor the new insights and healing.

Making Flower Essences, page 38

These are a few of my favourites, but you will have your own insights and understandings:

ELDERFLOWER ESSENCE
Helps us throw off old emotionally congested states, to move through old fears and bring clarity.

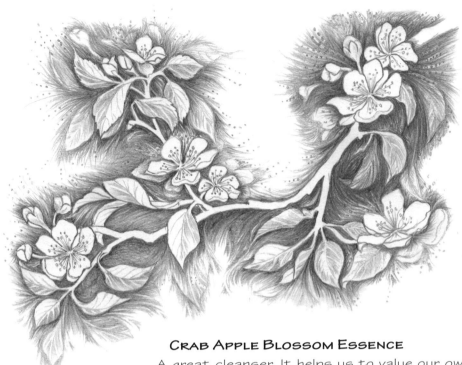

CRAB APPLE BLOSSOM ESSENCE

A great cleanser. It helps us to value our own abundance, count our blessings and to give generously of the love in our hearts.

OAK FLOWER ESSENCE

Helps us to stay earthed, balanced and solid in ourselves and to find our own inner strength.

ROWAN FLOWER ESSENCE

Strengthens our positive life energy and personal power. Brings a lightness of being and lifts the spirits.

Foraging for Edible Greens and Medicinal Herbs

Cleavers, Chickweed, Comfrey, Dandelion, Garlic Mustard, Hawthorn, Hops, Mallow, Mint, Mullein, Nettle, Red Clover, Salad Burnet, Sorrel, Yarrow

There are a lot of edible greens about at this time of year so as you walk about, keep an eye open for good places to forage. The plants I list here are the ones covered by this book but of course there are so many more,

Never leave home at this time of year without a few brown paper bags in your pocket or bag. The calico bags that are replacing our plastic bags are brilliant as foraging bags.

Only pick plants if there are a lot of them, otherwise decide to come back for a few seeds in the autumn and grow them at home next spring. Make a herb foraging map for your locality so that you can return to the same places again next year and you know where to find a herb if you need it. If you don't have time to make a map then at least jot down where you found the plants in your herb journal and look up what you can use them for. Dry them for future use or preserve them in alcohol, vinegar, honey, or oil.

Foraged edible greens can be chopped up and added to your food at the last minute or made into spinach mixes, which have many uses.

Foraging, page 17
Map Making, page 197
Edible Greens, page 140
Plant Reference Guide, page 249

THE WILD GARDENER

* The Wild Native Edibles – Chickweed
* Harvesting Herbs – First Crop
* Getting to Know Your Plants
* Plant-Pot-Clusters
* Guerrilla Gardening – Planting Out and Aftercare
* A Flash Mob

In this busy time find stillness in being with the soil, being earthed, bare feet on the ground. Find your own medicine outside your door. The plants will help you. When we let down our barriers and open ourselves to the plants, we are no longer separated and cut off from a dialogue with their healing energies.

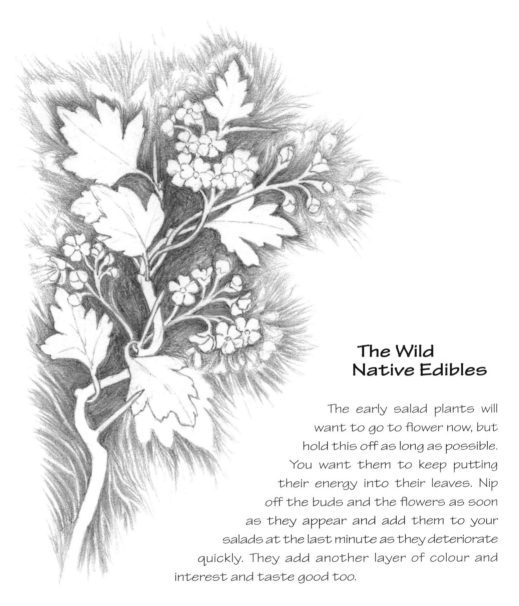

The Wild Native Edibles

The early salad plants will want to go to flower now, but hold this off as long as possible. You want them to keep putting their energy into their leaves. Nip off the buds and the flowers as soon as they appear and add them to your salads at the last minute as they deteriorate quickly. They add another layer of colour and interest and taste good too.

Eventually some of the plants will overwhelm you and you have to let them flower. Enjoy the flowers and then let them re-seed where they are, bending the seed-heads near to the earth to encourage them to fall in their own patch. They don't always stay there but the strays can get weeded out and eaten along the way. Alternatively keep your eye on the seeds ripening on the plants and shake them into brown paper bags when they are ready. Dry them well and store them in labelled envelopes for re-sowing later in the year.

CHICKWEED

Chickweed is a mainstay of my early salads but despite daily pickings of the tips it is desperate to flower now. I want to make sure I have lots of chickweed for the new season when it starts to grow again in early autumn. A trick of mine is to dig the plants up when they have finished flowering and are starting to go to seed. I put them back on the earth or in a large pot or two and put this out of the way to die back and let the seeds fall where I know where they are.

In August when the chickweed starts to grow again, I bring these pots back near the house to start cropping the succulent tips again. They transplant easily. Remarkably they will keep going until next spring as long as they are cropped frequently.

Harvesting Herbs – First Crop

The first herbs are ready to harvest now, just before they come into flower. Keep your eye on them so that you pick the optimum moment to harvest them.

As always take your time with this special moment. Cut them on a fine sunny day. Enjoy the plants in all their glory and perfection, and thank the plant before and after cutting the crop and take them inside to dry.

If you take this crop now, another crop will grow in a month. Leave the second crop to go to flower for the bees and butterflies and other winged insects that collect their nectar.

Drying Herbs, page 42

Getting to Know Your Plants

Spend time sitting amongst your plants to see what you can naturally sense about them from the way they grow, by where they choose to grow and what they look like. In the past herbalists would take all this into consideration when working with the healing properties of plants and this was known as the Doctrine of Signatures. Recognise when a plant is calling to you and spend time with that plant, appreciating all its wild beauty and intuiting how it makes you feel. Work with the same plant for a while and see the layers of understanding deepen.

Sit and draw the plant, whether you think you can draw or not. You are not doing this for the finished results, but to let yourself join with the plant. Feel the way the plant grows and how it lives in relationship to the other plants around it. Let go of your need for a formal picture, go wild, stop and restart at will, write on the picture, colour it in colours that you can sense rather than see, and represent its energy as flowing patterns or shapes.

Make a flower essence of any plant you are drawn towards and intuit what the plant has to tell you.

The Art of Seeing, page 152
Making a Flower Essence, page 38

Plant-Pot-Clusters

The seedlings you began growing in pots in the spring or last autumn should be coming through now and rather than do all that pricking out of the conventional gardener, I prefer to simply plant them out as Plant-Pot-Clusters. I remove the whole cluster of seedlings carefully from the pot and plant the whole lot as one item. This means the roots are less disturbed as they are transplanted, and they continue to grow in a clump. One or two of the strongest plants take over and become dominant.

Now and throughout the summer, make labels for all your herbs and native plants, and especially when you plant out seedlings. I make mine with pieces of slate, collected from beaches or from broken slate roof tiles. I write on them with a white correction marker pen, the ones that come in tubes that can be squeezed. It dries quickly and will last for a couple of years before it needs to be renewed. It gives you a reference point for where self seeded plants might appear the following spring or where perennials may shoot from.

Guerrilla Gardening – Planting Out and Aftercare

Check in on the areas you seed bombed earlier in the spring to see if any plants are growing. Sometimes germination is slow depending on the weather and success is not too high. Still it is fun to do and you may be rewarded with a clump of flowers blooming gloriously. Take bottles of water out with you to give any young plants a drink, especially if the weather is hot or dry.

Planting out established plants has a higher success rate and more visibly instant results. Grow plants especially for this, or dig up any plants from the garden to plant out. Again aftercare is so important and following through with weekly visits with water always helps plants to get properly established. Growing plants that can tolerate dry conditions and thrive on neglect also helps. This is where the native plants come into their own.

Plant out native plants as Plant-Pot-Clusters along footpaths and hedgerows by slitting through the soil with a good sharp pointed bulb trowel and slotting them in. These will also require extra aftercare and water while the plants get established so choose places you walk frequently and take pride in small successes.

Community guerrilla gardening projects can be great fun and there is something delightfully mischievous and wild edge about doing it. Being part of a guerrilla gardening group means that everyone works on the same patch or a variety of projects and helps and supports each other's work. Once even a small patch has been weeded, then regular visits are needed to keep it weed free and looking beautiful and well tended, so the more people willing to help the better. Talking to people about your group also helps to get new recruits, especially if a place begins to look better as a result of what the group is doing. Encourage friends to come along and join in.

Create an email-group or mobile phone group and use this network to let people know when and where you are guerrilla gardening, what plants are needed, to appeal for watering or compost etc.

A Flash Mob

A flash mob is an event organised by sending round a group text via mobile phones. It is used to let everyone know the time and place of a guerrilla gardening action, which would be improved by many helping hands, such as digging over a patch of ground in the spring, a mass planting up of an area with flowers or bulbs, or a tree planting event in the autumn.

KITCHEN MEDICINE

❀ Edible Flowers ❀ Drying Flowers ❀

❀ Flower and Leaf Tinctures ❀ Infused Herbal Oils ❀

❀ Herbal and Flower Syrups ❀ Flower Vinegars ❀

❀ Flower Cordials ❀ Flower Wines ❀ Tree Leaf Wines ❀

❀ Beech Leaf Gin ❀ Wild Salads from the Trees ❀

Nature is bursting with the life force now and everywhere there are wild salad greens, wild herbs and edible flowers to eat from the native wild plants and trees of this land. Many of these can be preserved for use later in the year.

Any dried herbs left over from the previous year need to be discarded now as the fresh herb becomes available. Sprinkle them round fruit bushes for an instant fertiliser and insecticide.

This is the time to harvest the tonic herbs, such as nettle tops, dandelion, cleavers, chickweed, when they are at their maximum power before they come into flower. This coincides perfectly with the need to weed them out to make way for more conventional crops. Eat them in your salad, add them to soups, dry them or make them into tinctures or oils.

Instead of conventional tea or bought tea bags, see what fresh herb teas you can create from the garden. Make the most of the wild plants and their vital energy. Look through the Plant Reference Guide on page 249 and see what might help you, or simply aim to build up your immune system with tonic herbs and immune system boosters.

Making Herb Teas, page 43

Edible Flowers

Chives, Cowslips, Dandelion, Elderflowers, Hawthorn flowers, Lady's Smock, Red Clover, Primroses, Violets

As the flower season begins, try using the flowers from edible plants in wild and inventive ways. They bring colour and beauty and an element of surprise! They deteriorate quickly so always add at the last moment. Sprinkle them over salads, and use them to decorate puddings, cakes and drinks. Make them into syrups, honeys, tinctures or if there are lots, then make them into a flower wine.

Drying Flowers

Drying flowers is a little trickier than drying leaves as they have to be dried quickly or they discolour. Therefore it is important to pick on a warm dry day and transfer to brown paper bags. These can be dried on the radiators or in the oven on a very low heat. Turn the flowers over with your hands frequently until they are dry.

Drying Herbs, page 42

Flower and Leaf Tinctures

Cowslip, Hawthorn, Lady's Mantle, Lady's Smock, Mint, Yarrow

These native plants are coming into flower at this time and can be made into tinctures for the home medicine cupboard. Tinctures last 3-5 years. Some you use occasionally, and some more frequently. Check your bottles and your herb journal to see what you have left, what you used often and what you think you might need in the coming year.

Read through the Plant Reference Guide, page 249, and see what you have got growing around you and what you anticipate you will need this year. Don't waste this precious resource, especially if you will weed them out anyway!

Write everything down in your herb journal – when you make your tincture, where you collected the plants from, their medicinal properties and anything else you intuit about the plant.

Making Tinctures, page 46
Plant Reference Guide, page 249

Infused Herbal Oils

Infused oils are simple to make and once made they will last for years. At this time of year they can be made from leaves or flowers.

This time of year make:

Elder Leaf Oil

For rashes, wounds, burns, sprains and bruises and a wonderful soothing oil for insect bites. It will also prevent insects from biting.

Dandelion Flower Oil

Rubbed into the skin for tired stiff joints and to loosen tense muscles.

Cowslip Flower Oil

Soothing to the skin and for sunburn.

Yarrow Oil

Make with the leaves and flowers. Use to stop bleeding, for inflammations and piles.

Making Herbal Oils (Macerations), page 53

Herbal and Flower Syrups

Dandelion flowers, Elderflowers, Red Clover, scented Rose petals, Mint, Rosemary and Lemon Balm

This is a delicious way for children to take their herbs and they can be drizzled on to porridge, ice cream, yogurt, as well as made into hot drinks. Make a note in your herb journal of what you have created, noting proportions and your methods.

Ingredients
1.15 litre (2 pint) glasses of leaves, flowers or fruit
0.57 litre (1 pint) glass of water
Sugar

Method One

1. Half fill a pint jar with leaves, flowers or fruit.

2. Cover with apple juice and let it steep for 24 hours, stirring occasionally.

3. Strain off the plant matter.

4. Bottle and label. Will keep for 3 weeks in the fridge.

Method Two

The more traditional method that will keep for many months.

1. Bring the plant matter and water to the boil, cover and simmer for 20 minutes and then strain through muslin.

2. Measure the liquid. For every 2 cups of juice add 1 cup of sugar and bring back to the boil in a clean saucepan. Stir and gently boil for about 10 minutes and pour hot into sterilised dark bottles.

3. Tighten the tops while hot. Label and date when cool.

Flower Vinegars

Good to make when you need to pick the flowers to prevent the plant from flowering but you don't want to waste the flowers. Simply pour some organic cider vinegar over the flowers. The herbal properties of the flower are preserved in the vinegar. Delicious to use in salad dressings and to drink hot with a spoonful of honey.

CHIVE FLOWER VINEGAR

At this time of year as the chive goes into flower, it is good to pick them so the plant gives its energy to its leaves. You will get another flower crop later. Chives are rich in iron. After a month strain off the beautiful pink vinegar, rebottle in a dark jar to preserve its colour, label and date.

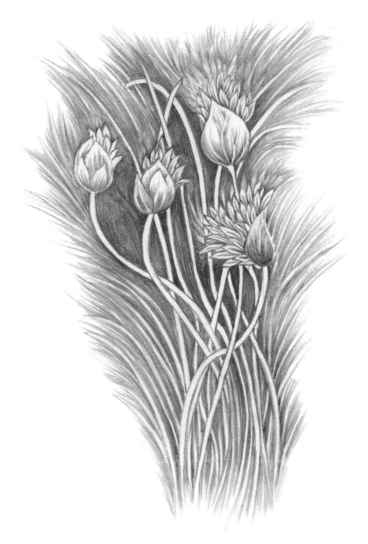

Flower Cordials

Broom, Dandelions, Elderflowers, Primroses, Cowslips, Red Clover, Sweet Violets, or Hawthorn flowers or any edible flowers

Create your own interesting creations using the basic recipe below. Dilute with water to drink, or pour neat over plain yogurt or other desserts.

ELDERFLOWER CORDIAL
As the elder comes into flower and fills the air with its heady scent, at least one batch of elderflower cordial or elderflower champagne must be made!

165

Add other perfumed flowers such as roses or aromatic leaves such as peppermint, to create new and interesting flavours or make with any of the flowers listed above.

Ingredients
12 large heads of elderflowers
3 lemons, chopped
600g (1lb) sugar
4.5 litres (8 pints) of boiling water
2 tablespoons (1oz) cream of tartar

Method
1. Put all the ingredients in a large bowl. Pour on boiling water and stir well.

2. Leave for 24 hours stirring occasionally.

3. Strain through muslin and pour into clean bottles.

4. Dilute to taste with still or fizzy water.

5. Will last a week or so in the fridge or can be frozen in plastic bottles for later use. (Don't fill the bottles to allow for expansion.)

Try adding oranges instead of lemons, and use a little less sugar.

Flower Wines

Elderflower, Dandelion, Hawthorn blossom, Broom, scented Rose petals, or any combination of edible flowers that you have a lot of and want to use

Cowslip wine was famously good, but of course you can only make it if you yourself grow an excess of cowslips. If using elderflowers or hawthorn flowers, gently strip them from their stalks using the fingers; for dandelions, cut off as much of the green stalk as possible; for broom pull the yellow parts from the green calyx, which is bitter. For roses, remove the petals from the plant without cutting the plant, so that the rosehips will grow.

Ingredients
2.3 litres (4 pint) of flowers stripped from their stalks or calyx
4.6 litres (1 gallon) of water
225g (8oz) minced or chopped sultanas
1.35kg (3lb) sugar
3 lemons
3 oranges
175ml (6 fl oz) cold black tea
1 teaspoon yeast

Method

1. Pour boiling water over the flowers and leave covered for three days. Stir every day.

2. Strain off the flowers. Bring the liquid to the boil adding the juice and finely grated rind of the lemons and oranges, sultanas, tea and sugar. Return to the bucket and when lukewarm sprinkle the yeast on top.

3. Cover with a tea towel tied round the top of the bucket with string and let this stand for a week.

4. Carefully strain off all the ingredients, and pour into a clean demijohn, and fit the fermentation lock. Bottle when fermentation stops.

Tree Leaf Wines

Oak, Birch, Beech or Lime leaves

All must be picked and made when the leaves are young.

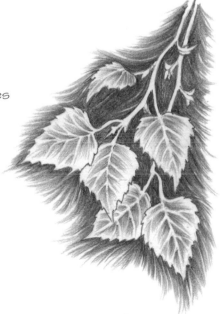

Ingredients
4.6 litres (1 gallon) of fresh young tree leaves
4.6 litres (1 gallon) of water
900g (2lb) sugar
2 or 3 oranges
1 teaspoon yeast

Method

1. Pour boiling water over the leaves, stir well and leave overnight.

2. Strain off the leaves and bring the liquid to the boil. Add the squeezed orange juice and finely grated rind.

3. Allow the liquid to cool to lukewarm, add the yeast and pour into a demijohn. Fit a fermentation lock and add water to the top of the lock to prevent the vinegar fly getting in.

4. When it stops fermenting, siphon the liquid from the sediment and either bottle the wine if it tastes good or return to a clean demijohn. Wine findings, pectinol or egg shells can be added to clear it if necessary.

Beech Leaf Gin

You will need a bottle of quality gin, a wide necked jar, sugar and fresh beech leaves.

1. Place the leaves in the jar and cover with gin, poking them down well so they are well covered.

2. Shake every few days for 2 weeks.

3. Strain off the leaves through a sieve, to reveal the brilliant bright green gin.

4. For every pint add 300g (½lb) of sugar, dissolved in 0.29 litre (½ pint) of boiling water. Mix the gin and sugar water and a good splash of brandy together and bottle up when cold. Ready to drink immediately, or will last for years if you can leave it that long!

Wild Salads from the Trees

Beech, Lime, Hawthorn, Elderflowers

Tree leaves are best eaten now while they are young. Use as the main ingredient for salads. Later when they are tougher they can be steamed gently and used in spinach type mixtures.

Gather and eat the sweet papery young leaves fresh from the tree. It is a short season so make the most of them. Make wild and beautiful salads using beech leaves (*Fagus sylvatica*), lime (*Tilia vulgaris*) and the first green shoots of the hawthorn trees.

Sprinkle salads with flowers from hawthorn and elder trees.

SEASONAL CELEBRATIONS

❀ Beltain

❀ Making a Foliated Headdress or Mask

❀ Making a Temporary Labyrinth

The sun is about to begin the final stage of its yearly cycle before it reaches the longest day and shortest night. All of life is on the move now, making the most of everything that this season has to offer. Our hearts are filled with wonder for the wild complexity and perfection of the natural world we are a part of.

This is a time of rapid growth when things can happen quickly. Initiate new ways forward that will help you develop and grow into the new holistic consciousness. As we each make the shift in our thinking, from self-interest to cooperation, from isolation into collective thinking, we pave the way for more change to happen, ever influencing those around us in subtle but profound ways.

Beltain
End of April – Beginning of May

Beltain is celebrated on or near the full moon or on May eve. It is one of the great fire festivals of our ancient past, when bonfires were lit on the hill tops and communities gathered around them, to stay up all night and see the summer in. It was a night for greenwood marriages, when couples would spend the night out in the woods together, celebrating their sexuality and love for life. It is a celebration of fertility and creation, the power of the life force to manifest and bring to life.

Traditionally Beltain is considered to be an edge place, a time in the Earth's cycle when the wild fecundity of life is so great that the edges blur, the veil between the worlds becomes thin and the spirits of nature are strong. This is personified as the spirit of the Green Man, the wild Earth spirit Herne and the wild spirit of nature that lives inside of us all.

It is a time to be open to the unexpected and to our wildest edges, a time to dare and to reach out for our most expansive visions, to fire up what we want to see happen, know that all things are possible. Great things happen when we are open to what we truly wish to manifest in life and when we are open to our own abundance. New experiences propel us forward and help us to grow new insights and understandings.

BELTAIN CELEBRATIONS

Included here are some ideas for connecting to the Earth, the seasonal energy, and your inner wisdom. Choose a couple of things to do, and be open to your own spontaneous inspirations of the moment.

For insights and overview about co-creating seasonal gatherings, see page 66

• At the full moon, decide to stay up all night with friends and enjoy those rich moments of transition between dusk and night, and night and dawn. Choose to walk to a place where this would be possible. Carry wood so that you can light a fire. Carry food and drink to share, sleeping bags and roll mats to sit on. If it won't disturb others, then drum together. Let words come through you as you weave your connection to the land and feel the Beltain energy grow within you.

• The Element of fire is celebrated at Beltain. It is the spark of life, the initiator, the transformer, activating whatever we give our energy to. What we choose to fire up now will come to life, continue, grow, and become active within us and in our lives.

If indoors, light a candle for each thing you wish to bring energy to in your life right now.

• Light an outdoor fire where there is room for people to get a bit of a run up and be able to jump the fire in the old tradition of Beltain. It is best built on the flat or slightly sloping downhill, but not uphill! As you jump the fire, call out what you most want to fire up. Jump again and call out what you leave behind – the things that might hamper this new growth. Pledge yourselves to the Earth as you jump, or to each other or a new direction. Be open to miracles happening at this fertile time!

• Make a pledge or vow to be of service to the Earth, to be part of her human support system, to take less of the endangered resources and to give more back by way of time, support and helping people to change their awareness and relationship with the Earth. Call out your pledges as you jump the fire.

• If it is not possible to jump the fire then light candles for what you wish to bring to manifestation. Write on pieces of paper what you let go of that might block this. Burn them in the candle flame and place in a metal bowl with a lid, or bury them in the ground.

• Pass round a basket of ribbons and each take three. As dawn approaches go for a walk. Look at the tree's flowers, celebrate the rampant life force of the land. Tie your three ribbons on a tree of your choice with three wishes: one for the Earth, one for yourself and one for your community.

• Celebrate and honour the great abundance of the life force, the raw energy of life, your sensual nature and your sexuality. Celebrate the fertility that comes from all unions. Name what you bring together and intend to manifest as you light candles.

• Trust in the power of generosity and the giving and receiving of love as a force for change in the world. Whatever we give our attention to will grow. Ask yourself what you will give energy to. We are our own source of power. All acts of generosity, and loving kindness will grow at this the most fertile time of the year's cycle. Write about these things in your journal.

• Gather round an outdoor fire and pass round a basket of dry sticks. What do you wish to let go of? What holds you back and drags you down? What negative feelings do you carry around with you and what negative stories do you tell yourself which block good things happening to you? Gather these insights into yourself and then let them go as you throw each stick in the fire. Call out what you let go of as you throw it in the flames. Give it power, strength and resolve. Burn many sticks if you have to!

• Another round of dry sticks can be passed round and thrown in the fire to fire up what you are thankful for in your life and what you wish to grow in your life.

• A change of heart will set you off on a new journey. Gather your boldness to begin so that you don't miss the opportune moment. Be prepared to move when the openings come. Act from the wild edge of your spontaneity and joyful zest for life. Gather nourishing intentions, foster loving kindness, feed yourself loving thoughts, words and food. Ask yourself what you want to grow in your life right now. Keep mindful of your intentions and lay the foundation stones for your future growth and the life you wish to live. Strengthen them every day by supportive actions and positive life-affirming thoughts. Choose what makes you happy, for here lies the source of our healing, our good health and our abundance. Write about your intentions in your journal and share with each other.

Making a Foliated Headdress or Mask

Headdresses or masks are traditional to wear for Beltain celebrations, to honour the beauty of the Earth and the beauty of each other.

For the headdress, make a simple circle the size of the head using pliable stems, and then weave in flowers and fresh greenery.

Making a Headdress, page 90

Making a foliated mask can be achieved by making a simple light willow framework and with the help of raffia or natural garden string, weave and tie in flowers and greenery. Tie leather thong, ribbon or garden string either side of your mask and tie at the back of the head.

Making a Temporary Labyrinth

Walking the labyrinth is traditional at Beltain. A labyrinth is always one continuous path in and out, without the false paths of a maze. The turning of the pathways facilitates the brain to switch from left brain to right brain, and to release spontaneous thoughts from the wild edge in between.

A temporary labyrinth can be made in a couple of hours using soil, sand, small stones, compost or bark mulch decorated with flowers.

Indoor labyrinths can be made out of cheap pouring salt, which is easily swept up at the end. Decorate with shells and stones and light up with night lights. Don't put salt outside on the earth as it will kill the vegetation.

FIVE RINGED LABYRINTH

This is quicker to create than the traditional seven paths, and is quicker to walk.

1. For a labyrinth that has 60cm (2ft) paths, the diameter will be approximately 6m (20ft) across. If you make the paths wider then the diameter will increase.

2. Begin by marking out five concentric circles with sticks or stones. Use a 60cm (2ft) measure-stick to measure the width of the pathways. Once these are all in place, check the diagram and decide where the entrance will be and what pathways need to be blocked off in relation to this. Again use pieces of wood or stones. In-fill with larger stones, sand or soil, more wood or bark mulch.

3. Using hazel stakes and ribbon makes a temporary labyrinth for events. You will need approximately 160 hazel stakes, each about 60cm (2ft) long, with one end sharpened; ribbon or material cut into long strips; or coloured wool. White ribbon looks amazing and shines in the dark. The hazel stakes are hammered into the ground plan and the ribbon, material or wool is wrapped around the stakes according to the plan. For safety, wrap the tops of the stakes with strips of material.

4. The labyrinth can be lit up at night by placing nightlights in jam jars along its pathways. Place something beautiful at the centre.

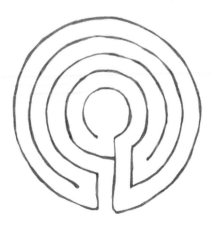

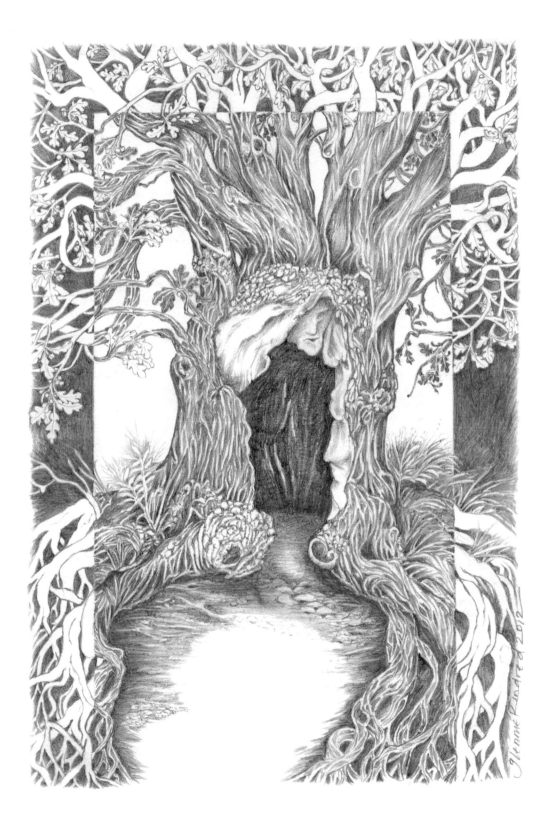

SUMMER'S
wild edge

June into July

This is summer's height, when the warmer longer days and late nights make it possible to spend more time outside, eat our meals in the garden, go for picnics and long evening walks, and generally make the most of this beautiful season. The world has turned green again as warm rains, sunshine and the increase in daylight bring rapid growth. This is the season of flowers, when it can seem like all of nature is in celebration of itself and its own wild beauty.

Take time off from your normal routines and get outside as often as you can. Give yourself to total appreciation of the natural world and the utter beauty and perfection of flowers. Fall in love with flowers, plants and trees. Fall in love with the Earth and the awesome perfection, wonder and beauty of the natural world.

This is a time of high manifestation and fertility. All energy is cyclic and is ever-flowing. Whatever we release into the flow determines what happens next and will eventually return to us – as all things are connected. Become aware of the powerful natural forces that are at work within you and around you, the powerful and subtle life force that is constantly forming and reforming depending on what we bring to the flow through our thoughts and feelings and actions. Strengthen your allegiance to the Earth. Find and act on all the ways that you can help nature regenerate and grow. The future is in our hands now, in this moment.

OUT ON THE LAND

❀ A Solstice Pilgrimage

❀ Breathing with the Trees – The Oak

❀ Restoring Balance

❀ Drawing and Painting with Natural Earth Pigments

❀ Making Flower Essences

❀ Foraging For Medicinal Herbs

Summer is the time to go on long trips to visit special places, to camp out, walk the land and connect to the Earth. Find trees to sit with and get to know, seek out native plants wherever you go, learn from them, learn about them and above all celebrate them. They are easy to identify this time of year as they come into flower. Carry a field guide around with you. Learn about their medicinal properties. You will be amazed what they can do and wonder how we have come to leave them behind! Share what you know about them to others. Talk to people about the importance of our native plants to the bees and the natural ecology of our land. See yourself as an ambassador for the Earth. Everything we do makes a difference and adds to the growing awareness of the interconnected whole.

A Solstice Pilgrimage

Plan a special trip out on your own for the Solstice. If you can go out on the day itself that makes it all the more special, but the power of the Solstice is there for at least a week either side of the actual date, so don't be put off by thinking it can only be celebrated at one specific time.

Visit somewhere that has power and significance for you and use this day as a review – to look deeper at some of the things that have touched you and shaped you in the last 6 months since the Winter Solstice. Celebrate all your achievements and especially how your relationship with the Earth has deepened. Look to the future and make a pledge to live with an even greater Earth-awareness. Explore what this might mean to you as you deepen the layers of understanding and insight that this brings.

For a real adventure and wild edge experience, sleep out on the land.

Alternatively plan a silent Wonder Wander with friends and enjoy the experience of being out on the land from dawn till dusk and the deepening that having a day in communion with nature brings.

Pilgrimages, Wonder Wanders and Vision Quests, page 15

Breathing with the Trees

Put aside time to be with trees. Find woods to walk in and walk with mindful open awareness of the trees and their different energies. When a tree calls you, then greet it with joy and value this experience. Place your back against its trunk or climb into the tree and spend time breathing deeply the oxygen rich air around the tree. Five minutes of deep-tree-breathing will bring many benefits to your body, filling your cells with life-giving oxygen and the air-born nutrients which the trees bring up from deep within the ground.

Listen to the song of the trees, the sound of wind in the leaves – different for each tree species and different at different times of the year and in different weathers. Allow the tree to help you slow down so that you can listen with your heart.

I often find myself crooning to trees; it seems to create connection at a deep subliminal level and moves me to open myself up to the subtle forces, the spirit of the tree and the edge of my wild self. It feels like the tree is singing through me sometimes.

Thank the tree before you leave, as this helps build personal and heartfelt connection. Our appreciation keeps our hearts open and paves the way for that wonder of wild edge phenomena – of having true friendship and relationship with trees.

THE OAK

Set out on a quest to find your nearest oak tree that you can sit with and learn from. The oak is linked with the Summer Solstice in folklore and legend as the doorway into the inner realms and the new cycle that is about to begin. Oak roots go deep into the ground to balance the heavy branches above. There is as much root below ground as branches above. This reminds us to keep the balance between all that we work and strive for in the outer world and like the oak, make sure that we anchor ourselves deeply into the Earth for our stability.

Restoring Balance

Nature slows us down, helps us to soften and restore our natural balance. At this time of year when we are often very busy it is essential to make time for walking in the green world, soaking up the beauty and letting ourselves simply be. When we remember to extend our senses we find there is so much more going on in the world around us than we realized.

Walking gets everything moving, not just on a physical level. It creates fluidity in the mind and frees up our thinking. Our inner intelligence also becomes engaged as our heart interprets the natural world around us and we become so much more alive to our whole selves.

As you walk become aware of your body and move in a way that is loose and flexible. Sense the Earth's power travel up from the depths of her and enter your body, so that you feel the Earth's strength running through you, and you feel it as your strength.

Lie on the Earth at every opportunity. Thank gravity and marvel at the Earth's perfection and beauty. Sit in natural hollows, out of the wind, find favourite trees to sit with or sit with your back against the Earth's living rock. Relax and breathe with the Earth so you can feel her power and feel yourself to be part of the vital life force of the land. Remember to look for places on your walks where you can take off your shoes and walk in direct contact with the ground or get your feet into natural water. See how invigorated and changed you are by this.

Barefoot Walking, page 14

Drawing and Painting with Natural Earth Pigments

While you are out walking, look for natural earth pigments and clays that will stain the page and have a go at drawing with them. Finding charcoal from the remains of fires is also a plus. Draw with your fingers and your own spit, draw or scratch through with a stick or a feather. The beauty of this is in the simplicity and the deep connection it brings.

You may also want to collect some of the earth and take it home for further experiments. When you get it home let it dry out and then grind it up in a pestle and mortar, or pound it to a powder with a stick or stone and store it in lidded jam jars. Label with the date and location. They can be used in ceremonies for marking faces and creating connection to a place. There is a wild magic in using earth in this way.

Try mixing the earth pigment with beaten egg white to thicken it. Paint on hessian, sail cloth or unbleached cotton with your hands or your feet as well as brushes. These can be lashed into willow or hazel circles or hung between sticks.

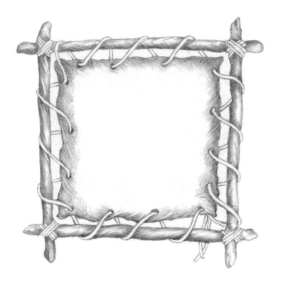

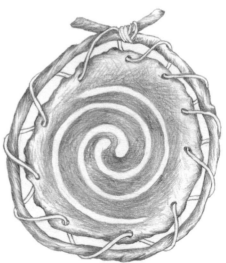

Making Flower Essences

Betony, Comfrey, Crab Apple Blossom, Dandelion, Elderflowers, Hawthorn, Lady's Mantle, Mallow, Mullein, Nettle, Red Clover, Rose, Self Heal, St John's Wort, Valerian, Vervain, Yarrow

With so many flowers at this time of the year, make yourself a flower essence kit, which is always at the ready to take out with you. In a dedicated bag wrap a small glass dish in a scarf or piece of cloth, a small glass bottle of spring water, one or two small dropper bottles half full of brandy, a small plastic jug, labels, a note book and a few crayons.

Flower essences are a simple way to tap into the essential energy of a plant. They can be used to energetically support a tincture or herb you are taking, or to help bring about an emotional shift to aid healing. They can also be made from non-edible plants, (especially if they keep calling to you).

For the Metaphysical Uses of the edible and medicinal plants listed above, see Plant Reference Guide, page 249
Making a Flower Essence, page 38

Foraging for Medicinal Herbs

Cleavers, Comfrey, Elderflower, Red Clover, Self Heal, St John's Wort, Hawthorn, Mallow, Hops, Rose petals, Mint, Mullein, Yarrow

This is the prime time for foraging for medicinal herbs just as they are coming into flower. Keep an eye open as you walk for where these plants grow in profusion. The ones I list here are the ones covered by this book but of course there are hundreds more.

Herbs are best picked and used fresh. They can also be picked for drying or tincture making. Gather herbs around midday on a dry sunny day. Don't gather when the plants are wet.

Make a herb foraging map for your locality so that you can return to the same places again next year and you know where to find a herb if you need it. If you don't have time to make a map then at least jot down the where you found the plants in your herb journal and take photos.

Foraging, page 17
Drying Herbs, page 42
Making Tinctures, page 46
Map Making, page 197
Plant Reference Guide, page 249

THE WILD GARDENER

❀ Harvesting Your 'Weeds' ❀ Edible Flowers
❀ Making Liquid Fertilisers
❀ Guerrilla Gardening – Caring For Neglected Corners

If you have a garden then now is the time to make the most of it. Think of your garden as an outdoor room. Move a table outside and eat and work outside, even when the sun isn't shining. If it is cooler, then wear a coat. If it's hot then take your clothes off and soak up the vitamin D from the sun. If it's wet, create an under-cover area. Take off your shoes whenever you can and enjoy direct contact with the Earth.

Move the tables and chairs around your garden according to the season and the position and intensity of the sun. Create morning or evening sitting and eating areas, put up screens for naked sun-bathing and create shaded areas, so you can be outside as much as possible. Create an outdoor fire pit, and invite friends and family to bring food to share and share the fire space. Locate it close to the house for ease of bringing out food and chairs. Moroccan stoves and fire dishes are moveable fires well worth investing in if you like to sit outside into the long summer evenings.

Drop the need to be only outside on fine days. Garden in the rain, in the early morning or into the half light of the evening.

Harvesting Your 'Weeds'

It is a full time job to keep up with nature's wild fecundity at this time of year and increasingly I am dropping my conditioned-need to have everything looking tidy in the garden. The garden becomes full of surprises as plants grow in unexpected places, form unexpected relationships and new plants arrive on the wind or via the birds.

Eventually all this wild fecundity will need to be weeded out to give conventional vegetables room to grow, but if your garden is made up of edible plants and medicinal herbs then these crops are utilised and turned into food and medicines. The numerous so-called weeds are cause for celebration as they are harvested, eaten, made into wine, ales, cordials, green smoothies, tinctures, herbal oils, pickled or dried. Nothing is wasted, and everything is valued. Anything left over goes in the compost. This is sustainability at its most immediate.

Edible Greens, page 140

Edible Flowers

Most of the edible leaves you have been eating since the spring will be desperately trying to flower now. Once the flowers form, then the leaves become bitter and inedible. You can eat the flowers of all the plants that you eat the leaves of, so the flowers become the next crop.

Pick flowers fresh just before you use them and add them to salads or as beautiful colourful garnishes. Use them for making any of the following for later use in the kitchen.

Flower Vinegars, page 164
Candied Flowers, page 188
Flower Cordials, page 165
Flower Wines, page 166

Always leave a few plants to flower, to enjoy their beauty and let them go to seed. Let them self-seed or collect the seeds to grow more plants next year.

Seed Collecting, page 225

Making Liquid Fertilisers

Make your own *effective* fertiliser brews from the comfrey and nettle plants you are clearing out at this time of year. Cut them off at the base so they can re-sprout and send up new leaves to add to spinach mixes or for herb teas later on. Lidded buckets and containers are worth getting for this purpose. Place them out of the way to mature in peace. Stir them frequently to help cut down the smell.

Method One
Chop up nettle, comfrey and red clover. Add seaweed and horse manure if you

have access to it. Half fill the bucket with plant matter and then top up with water. Stir well, cover and leave for 2 weeks, stirring frequently. Carefully pour off the liquid and bottle up in old water bottles.

Method Two

Mix one third well-rotted horse or chicken manure with two-thirds water. Stir well. Ready to use in a couple of days. Keep adding water to the manure left in the bottom of the bucket until you feel all the goodness is out and then spread anything left around the base of plants.

Method Three

Mix 5 parts water to 1 part fresh urine and use it to water the base of plants. This simple and effective fertiliser is ready to use immediately.

Guerilla Gardening – Caring For Neglected Corners

Look for small neglected corners you could make beautiful, perhaps in old churchyards or the site of a spring or well that is no longer used or visited. Look for ancient trees that may have once marked a special place. Decide to become a protector and guardian of this place and do a little wild-gardening, sensitively cutting back brambles if necessary and revealing what may be hidden. Only plant native plants here so that what you add is part of the natural native environment.

Check on other plants you have planted out previously and see how they are doing, making sure they are not getting swamped by grasses. Take bottles of water out with you for evening strolls and give them a water as they get established.

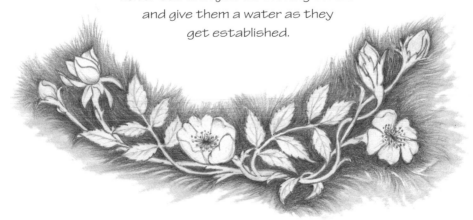

KITCHEN MEDICINE

❈ Drying Herbs for Future Use ❈ Drying Flowers
❈ Flower Tinctures ❈ Infused Flower Oils
❈ Herbal Honeys ❈ Candied Flowers

With the rich abundance of plants and herbs coming into flower, this is the main time for cutting and drying them for future use. Catching the right moment to pick plants and finding ways to preserve them for the winter months, creates an ever-deepening connection to the land and the seasonal cycles.

When we value and use the native plants in this way a whole new world opens up within us. We learn to make the most of what we have growing around us and not to waste nature's gifts. No longer passive observers of nature, we become engaged and thankful for the plants and their ability to heal and feed us. We become empowered by our knowledge and actively engaged in our own healing.

Our knowledge and confidence grows each year and is strengthened with each experience of restored wellbeing and our ever-deepening understanding of the interconnected web of life.

Cutting Herbs for Future Use

An awareness that I am cutting the plants off in their prime is always with me as I prepare to harvest them, so I totally appreciate them before I cut them and thank them for their gift of life and healing. This is not a job to rush, but to savour.

Sit a moment before picking to admire their beauty and perfection. Let your intuition roam and see what you intuitively understand about the plant at a subtle level. Look at its flowers and leaf shape, the way it grows and where it chooses to grow. There is much to learn about a plant at this point when it is at the peak of its power. There is more to the plant's healing properties than a text-book list of physical ailments. When you cut them yourself, thank the plant for its help.

Kitchen Medicine, pages 35-53

Drying Flowers

Betony, Elderflowers, Mallow, Mullein, Red Clover, Rose Petals, Self Heal, St John's Wort, Sweet Violets, Lavender

Drying flowers is a little trickier than drying leaves as they have to be dried quickly or they discolour. They can be dried in a very low oven or in brown paper bags placed in a warm dry airy place. Turn them over with your hands frequently to keep the air circulating. Don't over-pick and let some of the flowers carry on flowering, so that they mature and create seeds.

For most flowering plants it is true to say that the more you pick, the more you get, as the picking stimulates the plant to produce more flowers.

Drying Flowers, page 162
Herb Teas, page 43

Flower Tinctures

Betony, Chive, Elderflower, Mallow, Mullein, Red Clover, Rose petal, Self Heal, St John's Wort, Vervain

Tincture making is a quick and easy way to preserve flowers for future medicine.

Check the Plant Reference Guide at the back of the book for the medicinal uses of the above native plants that are in flower now. This will help you decide what you need to make for your medicine cupboard. They are all safe and effective medicines you can use with confidence and they cover a wide range of conditions.

Before gathering the flowers, take some time to sit and be with the plant, to appreciate the beauty of the plant and its life force and to thank the plant. Make the tincture as soon as you can after picking to preserve the vitality of the plant.

Write everything down in your herb journal so that your knowledge grows every year and every time you make and begin to use a new remedy.

Making Tinctures, page 46
For medicinal properties, see Plant Reference Guide, page 249

Infused Flower Oils (Macerations)

Self Heal, St John's Wort, Mallow, Mullein, Rose petal, Lavender, Marigold

Infused oils are simple to make, but only make small amounts at a time. They need to sit in the sunshine to infuse. They can be made with a good quality organic olive oil or sunflower oil but fine oils such as almond or jojoba, are more easily absorbed into the skin.

Making Herbal Oils (Macerations), page 53

SELF HEAL OIL
Make this excellent healing oil from the flower tops and leaves.

It is a major wound herb for cuts, sores, ulcers and piles. It will also aid and support the immune system and the adrenal glands. Add to massage oil and use as a foot rub.

ST JOHN'S WORT OIL
Pick the flowers around midday if you want your oil to go red. A wonderful healing oil, with antiseptic properties. Good for bruises, sprains, wounds, sciatica, shingles, backache, headache, rheumatic pain, burns, cuts, sores, varicose veins and ulcers.

N.B. See page 275 for when not to use.

MALLOW OIL
Make with the flowers and a few leaves. It is soothing and healing. Use for any skin problems or irritations, acne, burns, sunburn, sprains, muscular aches and pains. It will draw out a boil or a splinter. Good for insect bites, wasp or bee stings.

MULLEIN FLOWER OIL
Prized for dealing with ear-ache and ear infections. Also for any skin problems, acne, boils, bruises, sprains, muscular aches and pains, for scalds, burns and sunburn and for insect bites and stings.

ROSE OIL
Cooling to all hot conditions and good for the heart. It will strengthen your immune system and vital life force. Use highly perfumed roses such as *Rosa Gallicia* or

Rosa damascena, any highly perfumed garden rose or dried rose petals from a herbal supplier. Take the petals out of the oil after 1 week and replace with a second lot of petals. Do this several times to increase the scent.

LAVENDER OIL (*Lavandula officinalis*)

This not a native plant but it is worth making this wonderful soothing oil that will relieve sunburn, burns, insect bites and stress headaches.

MARIGOLD OIL (*Calendula officinalis*)

This is also not a native plant but well worth growing and macerating the petals in oil. It is excellent for dry chapped skin, 'gardener's hands', cuts, sores and babies' bottoms.

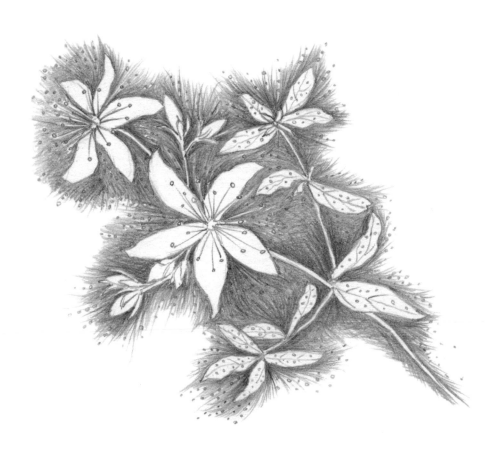

Herbal Honeys

Elderflower, Mint, Red Clover, Rose Petals, Vervain

Herbal honeys can be taken by the spoonful, added to yogurt, ice cream or fruit, or made into delicious drinks. They are great to make with children, helping them become active in their own medicine making! As always appreciate and thank the plants you use and send your thanks to the bees for making the honey.

Check the Plant Reference Guide for the properties of the plants.

N.B. Do not give honey to babies under 12 months.

Making Herbal and Flower Honeys, page 51
For medicinal properties, see Plant Reference Guide, page 249

Candied Flowers

Try Red Clover, Heartsease, Mallow, Rose Petals, Sweet Violets, Borage

This is an age-old way of preserving flowers for future use. It is a very relaxing and meditative thing to do.

Method
1. Remove the stalks and white bases from the petals.

2. Beat an organic egg white until foamy.

3. Dip each petal in the egg white and then in fine sugar.

4. Place on greaseproof paper on a cooling rack.

5. Cover with another sheet of greaseproof paper and leave in a very low oven with the door open until dry.

6. Store in airtight containers and use to decorate cakes and desserts.

SEASONAL CELEBRATIONS

❀ Summer Solstice

❀ Making a Medicine Bundle

❀ Making Medicine Bags

Everything is happening fast now. This is the height of nature's active power and an opportunity to make our every thought, emotional response, words and interests make a difference to those around us in our everyday lives and to those we meet. Share what you know and what you think. Change begins with you and me and in our many different communities. Change begins with the simple, the heartfelt and the joyful, and through activities that encourage us to be more open, more trusting and more willing to let go of the old ways.

Let us shine brilliantly like the sun at its height and celebrate being part of this worldwide movement for positive change. Stand up for what you believe in, consume less and when you do, consume ethically by giving your support to all the wonderful small businesses and products that are based on the same ideals, Earth-awareness and integrity as your own.

Summer Solstice
20th - 24th June

The Summer Solstice marks the longest day and shortest night of the year in the Northern Hemisphere. From this point onwards the days will shorten and the nights will lengthen until we reach the Winter Solstice once again. By marking the Solstices we acknowledge this beautiful flowing symmetry that brings balance to the natural world and into our lives.

The Summer Solstice is a moment to pause, to look back and celebrate all that we have actively achieved in the last 6 months since the Winter Solstice. It is an opportunity to take these achievements into our hearts and deepen our understanding of their significance and their potential to bring positive and beneficial change.

This is a transition moment, a recognition that a new cycle is about to begin, a moment to give thanks for the light and the dark, for both parts of our whole selves, inner and outer and the opportunity for transformation this brings.

SUMMER SOLSTICE CELEBRATIONS

Included here are some ideas for connecting to the Earth, the seasonal energy, and your inner wisdom. Choose a couple of things to do, and be open to your own spontaneous inspirations of the moment.

For insights and overview about co-creating seasonal gatherings, see page 66

• On Solstice morning climb high and face the north east to celebrate the rising sun and welcome the return of the dark cycle. If it is cloudy, sense the sun as it rises above the horizon and the day lightens. Give thanks for the balance of light and dark, outer and inner, active and receptive. Celebrate your achievements and all that you appreciate about the Earth and your life. Name these so that it is this contentment that you take with you into the new cycle.

• Go for a walk on Solstice morning and as you walk think about what you have achieved so far this year both for yourself and with your deepening journey with the Earth. Ask yourself what do you choose to do now that will help to strengthen your new ways forward? Look for a natural feature in the landscape that you can use as a doorway, such as two trees. Pause at the threshold and gather into your heart all that you celebrate about the last 6 months and as you step through the doorway, and name what you take into the new cycle.

• Gather with friends on Solstice Eve. Locate a high point from which you will be able to see the sun as it rises in the north east. Ask everyone to bring food and drink to share, but no alcohol as it deadens the senses and changes the atmosphere. Ask everyone to bring some firewood for the fire. Stay up all night and enjoy being out under the night sky. As dawn approaches and the sun appears over the horizon celebrate the sun in fine style with drumming and wild crowing! Take off your shoes and dance on the land. Let your heart expand with your love for life! Share breakfast together and go for a walk afterwards.

• Decide to have a day out on your own on the Solstice. Make a pact with yourself that you will *go whatever the weather!* Set the alarm for 3.30 am, which means you will be up before it is light. Light a candle and let your eyes adjust to the gentle half light. Have water and light food packed the night before so that all you need do is fill a flask, eat a simple breakfast and get outside quickly to enjoy the special atmosphere that only being out this early brings.

• Find a place that faces north east and watch the day break and hopefully the rising sun. Give thanks for all the wonders of our beautiful Earth and the miracle of our being here right now at this important transitional time. Pledge your allegiance to the Earth and name your new intentions for the new cycle.

• Somewhere near the Solstice, put aside a day for yourself. Treat yourself to a retreat day, and get away from all your normal jobs and routines. Plan a trip somewhere special to you. Spend as much of it as possible outside in mindful communion with the Earth. Pay special attention to your relationship with each of the five elements. Recognise when certain plants and trees are drawing you towards them and be open to the gifts and insights they bring. Write about this in your journal.

• Summer Solstice celebrates the return of the dark, the inner cycle. Celebrate those vital hidden parts of yourself, often forgotten or undervalued, such as your imagination, your intuition, your instincts and your feelings and all the things that help you to grow from the inside out. Name them and give thanks. Acknowledge your changing relationship to the dark as old fears give way to trust and a more balanced perspective.

• Look for a stone you are attracted to while out on the land. This becomes your Solstice Stone. Hold it as you meditate and contemplate this great turning point in the year's cycle. How will you make space in your life for inspiration from within? Use the stone to anchor your understanding and resolve.

• Gather with friends for a Solstice gathering and ask everyone to bring food and drink to share and crystals for a shared crystal basket. Sit in a circle and pass the basket around the circle. Each takes a crystal with thanks for the Earth. Share with each other what you celebrate about your life right now. Later take the crystal to a special place on the land and bury it, declaring your allegiance to the Earth.

• Summer Solstice is a moment of pause between the end of one cycle and the beginning of the next. Reflect on what you have achieved since the Winter Solstice, and what you have learnt from this part of your journey. Share this with each other and write in your journal.

• What old beliefs are you willing to leave behind? Look for where you become disconnected from nature and the Earth. What new intentions will help you move forwards? Write in your journal and share your insights with each other.

- Recount to each other the wild and outrageous things you did when you were younger. Where is this part of you now? How can you celebrate this wild part of yourself today? Make a pact with yourself to step more fully into your wild power, to have fun and enjoy these aspects of yourself. Tap into your wild zest for life, the wild fire of your passion, your love for life and for the Earth.

Making a Medicine Bundle

A medicine bundle is a way of seeking and gathering towards yourself the personal teachings you have received from the plants and trees.

1. Spend some time gathering together a small piece from each of the plants that have been your greatest teachers this year. Thank the plants.

2. Lay them out in front of you and name each understanding gained. Write in your journal. Seek the overall teaching that their combined strength gives you. This is the medicine of your medicine bundle.

3. Bundle them together by holding them against a piece of silver birch bark to represent the new beginnings that will grow from this moment. Wrap them all together with raffia, grasses or ribbon affirming the medicine of the plants, the teachings received and what you take forward into the new cycle.

Later this can be returned to the Earth or left at a significant place with your thanks for the wisdom gained.

Making Medicine Bags

Small medicine bags are worn around the neck and are used to carry something of significance whose energy or medicine brings protection or strength to the person who wears it. It may represent a teaching or medicine being worked with, a reminder, a talisman. Contents are usually natural but there are no rules. You might include herbs, a piece of wood or bark from a tree whose teachings are significant, a crystal, a stone, a piece of animal or bird bone, something found at a special moment or something from a place that is special to you. The contents of a medicine bag can be changed when it feels right, when a new medicine presents itself, or when the medicine of the bag is no longer relevant. A new medicine bag is made for a new beginning.

The old medicine bag and its contents are honoured and thanked. It may be saved as a reminder of your journey or buried in the earth with due ceremony.

A larger medicine bag is called the shaman's bag or crane bag and traditionally would hang from the waist – although I prefer a shoulder strap as it is easier for travelling. This is your mobile medicine chest and contains your bags of herbs and bottles of tinctures, elixirs and oils. It could include smaller medicine bags that group different herbs together that do a similar job, such a wound herbs, digestive herbs, herbs for colds or coughs etc. Use a system of colour-coded threads for easy identification. As dried herbs will only last a year and berries and roots for 2 years, the contents of the bags are revised every year and new herbs found to replenish dwindling stocks.

Method One
Making a Circular Bag
1. Cut a circle out of chamois, leather or other tightly woven cloth by drawing round a template of choice, anything from a small bowl to a large plate depending on the size and use of the medicine bag.

2. Cut or poke small holes around the outside of the circle.

3. Cut a long piece of leather thong or plait together some embroidery threads or wools to make a length, and thread this through the holes.

4. Decorate with coloured threads, embroidered or painted symbols, beads or anything else of significance.

Method Two
Making a Folded Medicine Bag
1. Decide on the size you wish your medicine bag. Fold a piece of chamois, leather or other tightly woven material in half, with the fold at the bottom of the bag for extra strength. Cut the sides to the shape you want.

2. Sew up the sides with strong leather thread.

3. Decorate with coloured threads, embroidered or painted symbols, beads or anything else of significance.

4. Cut or poke small holes around the top and thread with a length of leather or plaited threads or wool.

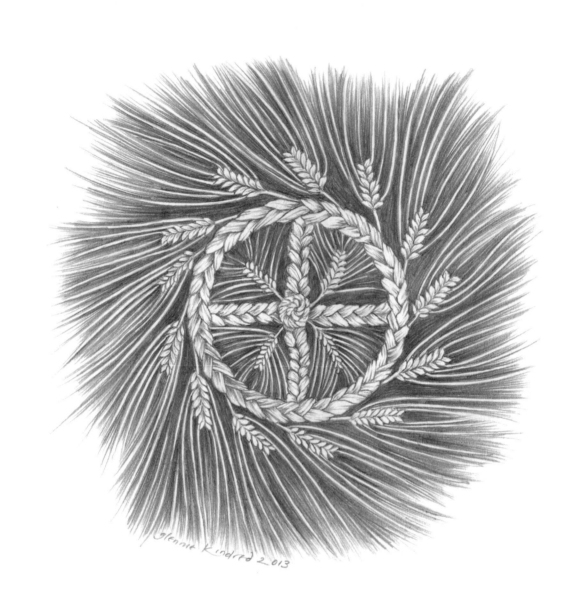
Glennie Kindred 2 013

on the edge of AUTUMN

July into August

Seed heads are starting to form, fruit is beginning to swell, mornings can start misty, thick with dew, and there can be a nip of cold at night. But for all this it is still summer and this is a time of holidays, festivals, living outside, camping out and summer nights spent with friends around outdoor fires. The feel-good factor abounds especially when the sun shines, as we enter this last phase of summer with an awareness that it won't last forever and autumn is on its way.

This is the time of Lammas, a time of plenty, when in the ancient past the tribes would have travelled to great clan gatherings to meet up with friends and family. In our more recent past, communities would have celebrated the great gathering in of the grain harvest. We too feel the pull to get out and about while we still can, travel, walk the land, visit friends, gather at festivals and community events.

It is a prime time for us to share ideas, our enthusiasm and passion for Earth awareness and living lightly on the Earth. We can each be a power-house of positive change in the world, inspiring ourselves and others to make the shift into a holistic life-view and work together for the common good and for the good of the Earth.

OUT ON THE LAND

❀ Jaunts and Adventures ❀ Map Making
❀ Time Alone ❀ Libations and Offerings
❀ Foraging – Early Fruit and Hazel Nuts

Throughout the land are many ancient trackways, ridgeways, hollow-ways, portways and other 'ways' that were once used by travellers and are still there to be followed. There are trade routes and packhorse routes that give us a glimpse of the lives and history of the past. They can lead us to forgotten beautiful places, hidden valleys, springs and wells, caves, hill forts, earthworks, Bronze and Iron Age burial mounds and settlements, and places where industry once flourished and nature is reclaiming.

Using an ordnance survey map find your way into the complex of footpaths and smaller lanes. Find places where the grass has grown high and the wild flowers are still growing. Collect a few seeds along the way. You don't need many if you grow them at home in a pot. Later when you have established a patch at home you can plant them back out to create new wild flower edges for the future.

When it is warm enough, throw off your clothes in wild abandon, lie in the long grass, go wild swimming and skinny dipping. Let the sun warm and brown your naked skin. Walk barefoot, in contact with the Earth, whenever you can.

Jaunts and Adventures

Have your day bag packed and at the ready for early morning jaunts and adventures. Add last minute drinks and food and surrender to the call of the natural world. Make the most of the long sunny days, plan picnics and days out on the land, with friends or alone. If you walk with friends, agree to have some silent time so that you can admire and make connection to nature and not just walk and talk through it.

Drop your fear of walking alone and venture out to wander where your intuition takes you. Carry an ordnance survey map of the area as a safety-net if you fear getting lost. Take off your watch. Watch the sun and become aligned to the directions and sun-time.

Visit your nearest large forest and learn to navigate by significant trees. You may get lost for a while and have experiences that require you to use your instincts and your knowledge and survival skills that let you know both you and the wild are very much alive. It's a good idea to let someone know where you are going if going alone.

Go for walks high in the mountains, where you have to keep your wits about you and keep an eye on the weather and your footing. Again, if you go alone, let someone know where you are going and check in with them when you are back.

Travel into gorges and gullies and observe the microclimate and the flora and fauna this supports. Spend time with wild gushing water or sit peacefully with the mesmerising power of the sea. There is so much to experience and see in this varied and beautiful land of ours!

Learn how to be still and silent. Push your senses to their wild edges. Look closer at the incredible detail of a flower or leaf, a butterfly's wing or a beetle. Absorb the shape and feel of the land, sense the forces that created it, the layers of history within it. Learn to recognise plants and trees by their smell. Listen to the sounds of nature, the call of a spring as the water surfaces, the voices of streams and waterfalls, the leaping of fish, the calls of the birds and animals… Feel your own wild edges expand, create connection, talk to plants, trees and birds and be open to communication from them. There is so much to experience when we slow down and open ourselves to this interconnective world we are part of.

Map Making

Once when travelling in Morocco, we met a map-maker. He arrived in the community where we were staying, and unrolled his hand drawn maps. They were a bit like the maps found in the inside of Tolkien's *Lord of the Rings*, with mountain ranges, villages, trees, springs and oasis' drawn in a semi symbolic style. His technique was to first climb to the highest point and transfer what he could see to his map. Later he walked the land and refined his map. He worked in pencil first and then went over it with ink when he was happy with it. He had arrived there because he was going to climb the mountain there and complete another part of the map he had of the area.

This process of building up a local map, drawn by hand and added to over the years as more things are discovered, is a joyful project to begin this time of year. It is creative and connecting and of course great to do with children. It helps anchor you in your locality and brings an awareness of the history of human life as it affects the landscape. It can be added to over the years and becomes part of your own history and family history. It doesn't have to be to scale, and can be refined and redrawn whenever you choose, so that it is always work-in-progress, always evolving.

Build your local map up on a series of A4 size pieces of paper. Use a good quality sketchpad for this so the paper quality is robust. Alternatively you can make a large wall-map by sketching or tracing off the details from your A4 maps.

Scanned or traced copies from previously drawn maps can be taken out with you and added to. Remember to date them as each season reveals new things. Keep all the copies you make, as there may be things on there that you come back to.

If you want to create a more specific map then trace off the main lanes, rivers, streams, hills etc from an ordnance survey map. Make a few copies of this basic map for taking out with you and then add in your finds. When you get home add the information to a main master copy.

Include the old local names for places as well as creating your own names that reflect your own experiences there. Add springs, brooks, rivers, copses and woods, footpaths, lanes, boundaries, ruins and any anomalies and features you notice. Mark in and name significant trees and hedgerows and where autumn fruits can be gathered. Mark on the places where you notice native plants growing, what time of year they are flowering or seeding. Your map can be used as a reference point in the future, especially useful if you are foraging wild food, need a plant for medicine, want to collect seeds or plant out native plants.

Time Alone

Don't be afraid to spend time on your own. Gift yourself time to think, muse and daydream, and simply find enjoyment in your own company. Set out to walk locally, taking a journal to write in, water to drink and food to nibble. Find your sense of contentment in yourself and the landscape. Whether in a town or countryside, there are always out of the way places to be found, trees to sit with and places where you feel comfortable to rest in.

Walking alone is a call to be bold, to move through old fears and find your confidence in yourself and with your relationship with the land. After a few trips your fears will fall away and you will feel exhilarated with a wild power and sense of freedom! Enjoy the sweet pleasures of reflection and connectivity. Extend your senses and awareness to see just how far you are able to communicate with the natural world around you. You need to be on your own to have your own experiences and to reach your own understanding of this.

Singing and crooning to the land is something I do when walking alone. This is no idle or nervous humming, but a way of making connection through sound. It is completely natural because I do it without thinking. I have done it all my life and I remember doing it as a child. It helps me slip into a meditative receptive place. It feels somehow primitive and ancient, a wild edge of my uninhibited self.

Make a walking stick to take with you as companion and friend. It has many uses besides the obvious one of helping keep you steady on rough ground.

Finding and Crafting Your Own Staff or Walking Stick, page 215

Libations and Offerings

A libation or offering is an ancient practice but is still very much alive today especially amongst the seafaring communities and amongst people who travel and those who live close to the land. A libation or offering acknowledges our openness to the interconnected web of life and powerful forces that also part of us, such as the elements, the spirits of place and the land, our guardians and spirit guides, and the ancestors. It is a giving something back, a giving of thanks or asking for a blessing, a safe passage, safe journey or protection. It can be totally personal, something you do alone, or as part of a bigger ceremony.

A libation is usually a liquid offering such as spring water, wine, oil, an alcoholic spirit, or milk, although it could be a cup of tea if it is offered in a heartfelt giving of thanks.

Offerings are usually grains, flowers, seeds, herbs or food of any kind. Offerings can also be a gift of soil, collected from sacred or significant places, unusual or special stones, crystals, shells, bones, feathers and other natural things. Water from different springs, stones or soil from different places and geodes cut in half can be used to connect places together. Offerings can also be burnt, such as the burning of herbs and incense.

When walking the land, it may come to you as you drink and eat your food, to share a little in thanks for all that the Earth provides for you. It may also be something you plan to do as part of a pilgrimage or vision quest. Make a special medicine bag for this and carry a small glass bowl for water.

Making Medicine Bags, page 192

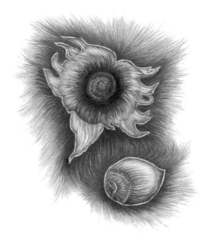

Foraging - Early Fruit and Hazel Nuts

This is the beginning of the fruit season, so keep a look out for where you will be able to gather fruit when it ripens. Blackberries, crab apples, rowan berries, haws and rosehips all begin to ripen now, especially in sunny spots. Elderberries and sloes come later. A plastic tub in your day bag is a must this time of year!

The purple fruit of the bilberry, sometimes known as blaeberry or whortleberry (*Vaccinium myrtilis*), ripen now between July and September and provide a tasty snack while out walking. It is a native shrub found on moors, mountains and in woods. Bilberries can be collected and brought back to add to garden fruit or dried for winter stews.

Hazel nuts are collected August to September. You will need to keep an eye on them and judge the moment to forage them before the squirrels collect them all and hide them away. Usually the first nuts to fall are the ones the tree has rejected and often don't contain any nuts. Pick them fresh from the tree, but not when they are too green. Find a flat stone and a striking stone and crack them open in this timeless way.

THE WILD GARDENER

❋ First Seeds ❋ Growing Cowslips, Primrose and Violets
❋ Winter Salad Plants ❋ Painting with Plant Pigments
❋ Cutting Back and Making Compost
❋ Marking Trees to be Moved ❋ Native Tree Seeds
❋ Guerrilla Gardening – Looking After Trees
and Community Celebrations

These are the heydays of summer, when garden crops are being picked and brought to the table. Early fruits are ripening in the garden now too, providing early morning foraging trips outside for breakfast fruit feasts. At this time of year more meals are eaten outside in the garden and any an excuse for an evening bonfire must be acted upon!

If you cut the first crop of herbs in early June, they will have re-grown now and be coming into flower. Leave the second crop for the bees and pollinators who love them.

This is the season of the native flowers. If you have grown them for medicine they will need to be picked now. If you have excess then enjoy their wild magic and pick glorious mixed posies to bring into the house or give to friends.

First Seeds

Cowslips, Cleavers, Corn Salad, Primroses, Salad Burnet, Violets, Winter Cress

The first seeds of the early spring plants are beginning to ripen now. Bend them gently over to encourage self-seeding where you want them to fall, or keep an eye on them and gather them when they are ready.

Spread them out on paper and sort through them, discarding any that do not look perfectly formed. Let them dry thoroughly in labelled brown paper bags before storing them in labelled envelopes in a cold dry place for the winter or sowing in the autumn.

Seed Collecting, page 225

Growing Cowslips, Primroses and Violets

1. Collect the seeds August to September when they ripen and sow immediately so that winter dormancy doesn't set in.

2. Use a good quality peat-free seed compost in deep pots to avoid the compost drying out. Thoroughly soak and then sprinkle the seeds on the surface – the seeds need light to germinate.

3. Spray with water to soak the seeds and put the whole thing in a plastic bag and tie up. Germination happens about 4-6 weeks later.

4. When the first true seedlings appear, plant them out in peat-free multi-purpose peat-free compost again, put the pots in partial shade and keep them well watered if necessary. Plant the young plants out in the spring.

Winter Salad Plants

Chickweed, Corn Salad, Lady's Mantle, Wintercress

Edible native plants are beginning to reappear and can be transplanted to dedicated beds or into pots near the house. I put them in with tomatoes or cucumbers, and when these die back in the autumn, a fine crop of native edible plants for the winter and spring remains. Start cropping chickweed now, adding it in with your salads, or grazing while passing; this ensures the plants don't get straggly and that they thicken up.

Painting with Plant Pigments

Have a little fun in your garden and see what plants you have that will make coloured marks on paper. Roll a juicy green leaf into a tight tube, rolling and squeezing it between the fingers to bruise the plant and get the juices flowing. Spitting on it helps too. Rub it on the paper and make a simple pattern. Then try this with flowers, which will bring other colours as well as surprises as their pigment is often not the colour of the flower.

Leave as it is or do some creative pencilling over the top or write the names of the plants near or on the colours once dry.

A lovely thing to do on a lazy day in the garden and of course children, and the child in all of us, delights in its simplicity.

Cutting Back and Making Compost

Eventually the wild edges have to be tamed at this time of year. Borders need tidying up and cutting back, so that new growth can begin again. Hedges need cutting back so that they don't become trees, and this is the ideal time now that the birds have finished nesting. This is the perfect excuse to make lots of different piles of compost matter.

Having lots of good quality compost is one of the mainstays of growing organically so it is worth putting time and energy into it. The green plastic compost bins are handy containers, especially in a small garden and are good for kitchen waste (no cooked food as this will attract rats), layered with plant matter, cardboard, rotted leaf mould and horse manure if you have a source of it. Our own urine will help the compost to activate it, so it's worth collecting it by your preferred method. A must-do for every wild gardener!

There are many native plants that I don't put in the compost bins. The roots of invasive weeds are burnt on the bonfire but other wild native plants are thrown under trees, along the hedge bottom and in the dark corners of the garden to feed the plants as they break down.

Hedge and tree trimmings break down more slowly, and can be made into rough piles along the wild edges. These provide places for wildlife and insects to live in. Old piles can be broken up this time of year if they have got too big and firewood and fire lighting sticks salvaged, dried out and stored for the winter. It does disturb a lot of insect life, but at this time of year they scurry about and re-house themselves quite easily. It's better now than doing it later when they need secure homes for the winter.

Marking Trees To Be Moved

Trees are a precious resource and not to be wasted, especially our native trees, many of which are fruit and nut bearing and edible. Now is a good time to mark any native tree seedlings that have self-seeded in your garden or near vicinity that will need to be moved in the winter. This is done now while you can identify them.

Tie on a label, write on a piece of slate with a white-out marker, or if you know your native trees, and don't need to label them, then simply tie a ribbon or piece of bright wool round them. Wool can also be colour-coded for different tree species. The trees can then be dug up in the autumn when their leaves have fallen and moved into the hedges or potted up until they are large enough to be planted out.

Native Tree Seeds

Alder, Ash, Blackthorn, Crab Apple, Elder, Hawthorn, Hazel, Holly, Oak, Rowan, Silver Birch

Extract the ripe seeds first, cleaning them off in water if necessary. Mix the seeds with a 50/50 mixture of peat free compost and sand and then scatter the mix fairly thickly onto a labelled holding bed or into labelled pots. Protect from rodents with fine mesh if necessary. In the spring see if any have germinated and pot up. Some tree seeds take two years to germinate.

Guerrilla Gardening –
Looking After Trees and Community Celebrations

Check in on all the plants or trees you have planted out this year. Tidy up around them and keep the base of young trees clear of strangling grasses. Take bottles of water out with you to water them in dry weather. This is very important in their all-important first year, especially if they were planted in the spring. They need the winter now for their roots to become deeper and more established.

If you have been guerrilla gardening with a group then make sure you have a community celebration to mark your achievements, however small they may seem. There are a lot of setbacks and disappointments to guerrilla gardening, especially in the early stages but there are always things to celebrate, lessons learned, new strategies to be discussed for the coming months and plans to be made for next year's projects.

Collect everyone's mobile number so that you set up a mobile guerrilla gardening group. This means everyone can let each other know when and where they are going to guerrilla garden, what they are doing or planning to do, and ask for help with clearing, planting or watering. Working together achieves more.

Flash Mob, page 160

KITCHEN MEDICINE

❀ Making Tea Bags ❀ Making Bath Bags
❀ Making a Herb Pillow ❀ Fruit Wine
❀ Fruit Vinegars ❀ Hops – Hop Beer
❀ Making Dark Storage Jars

There is much to process this time of year. Many plants are coming into flower and reaching the optimum time to pick them, to dry for winter use and make into tinctures and elixirs. The time of the first fruits begins and opens up a new set of possibilities.

Making Tea Bags

The herbs you picked last month will be dry now and you can enjoy making your own herbal tea blends. This is such a joyful alchemy and not only do you create a blend that is honed to what you need, but also to the tastes that you like and enjoy. Add small amounts of the aromatic herbs to the main medicinal herbs to create nice tastes. Try adding lemon verbena or lemon balm to calming blends; or rosemary, or peppermint to more stimulating blends.

Method

1. Cut lots of rounds of light muslin – about 10cm (4in) across. Use a dish or plate to draw round.

2. Put a teaspoon of the dried herb or herb blend in the centre.

3. Tie up with a cotton string or thread.

4. Store in a dark jar or brown paper bags as light will destroy their herbal properties.

5. Make as an infusion by pouring boiling water over the herb and covering. Drink hot or cold.

Infusions, page 44

Making Bath Bags

These are made in the same way as teabags but bigger. Mix combinations of herbs together depending on whether you wish to have a calming or stimulating bath, herbs for tired muscles etc.

1. Cut circles of muslin approximately 18cm (7in) across. Draw round a large plate.

2. In the centre place about 3 teaspoons of dried herbs.

3. Gather up into a bundle and tie round with coloured threads, wool or natural string. Leave long threads so that you can hang them over the hot tap. Colour codes could represent each herb added. Write this in your herbal note book.

4. Place in a jug of boiling water and let it steep for 10 minutes before adding the liquid and the bath bag to your bath.

Absorbing Herbs Through the Skin, page 52

Making a Herb Pillow

Betony, Hops, Elderflowers, Hawthorn flowers, Mullein, Chamomile, Lavender

Herb pillows are filled with dried herbs and flowers that are very calming and help you sleep.

Method
1. Fold a piece of cotton material approximately 30 x 30cm (12 x 12in) in half and sew up two sides.

2. Fill with dried herbs and press down until it feels a comfortable amount and then sew up the third side.

3. Slip into the pillow case of your normal pillow.

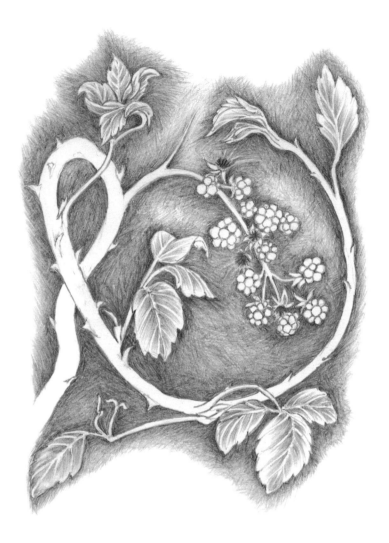

Fruit Wine

Blackberries, Crab Apples, Elderberries, Haws, Rosehips, Rowan

Wine making is a great alchemy, a way of using and preserving fruit and the herbal qualities stored within them. Fruit wines are usually the most successful wines, especially if there has been a good amount of sun to ripen and sweeten the fruits. Try mixing fruits with flowers, garden fruits with hedgerow fruits and adding herbs. Be inventive and creative and when you open them in 2 years time there will hopefully be surprises and delights in store. If not you can always use it for punch or in cooking or create blended mixtures later on!

There are many recipes for fruit wines but a basic recipe can be adapted, different fruit substituted, varying amounts of sugar or extras added. Keep good records of your creations so that you can repeat them another year if you make a good one. Fruit wines vary from year to year depending on the sweetness and ripeness of the fruit, the amount of autumn sunshine or rainfall, so it is never an exact science.

Try and keep a wine for 2 years after bottling it up before drinking it with due ceremony; a toast to the fruit and to the Earth and to the person who made it. If you can keep back one bottle from each batch to drink many years later it improves hugely and there is something poignant and rather special about looking back and remembering a year long gone.

This is a basic fruit wine recipe for 1.35kg (3lb) of fruit:

CRAB APPLE AND BLACKBERRY WINE

>1kg (2lb) ripe crab apples
>450g (1lb) blackberries
>l orange
>1.35kg (3lb) sugar
>3 litres boiling water
>1 teaspoon of yeast

1. Rough chop the apples into a plastic bucket and add blackberries, the orange peel and juice. Pour on the boiling water and cover with a tea towel tied round the top of the bucket.

2. Let it steep for three days, stirring daily.

3. Strain off the fruit. Heat up the liquid and stir in the sugar until dissolved.

4. When lukewarm stir in the yeast and pour into a demijohn. Fit a fermentation lock and leave in a warm place until it stops fermenting. Siphon off into wine bottles and cork.

Fruit Vinegars

Another way to preserve fruit is to pickle them in vinegar.

BLACKBERRY OR RASPBERRY VINEGAR
Rich in vitamin C and drunk with hot water in the winter to ward off a cold.

1. Cover 225g (8oz) of blackberries or raspberries with 370g (13 fl oz) of wine or cider vinegar. Leave for 4 days in a cool place, stirring occasionally.

2. Strain off the fruit, pour the vinegar back into the bowl and add another 225g (8oz) of blackberries or raspberries. Cover and leave for another 4 days.

3. Strain the vinegar through a jelly bag or muslin and measure it.

4. Put into a saucepan, add an equal weight of honey to vinegar, and gently bring to the boil. Simmer for 5 minutes and skim well. Pour into a jug, cover with a folded tea towel and tie round it with string. Leave for 24 hours and then bottle in dark bottles.

Hops

Hop flowers should be dried as soon as they come into flower. Catch them before they go brown and hang them in brown paper bags where it is warm and dry until they become papery. Alternatively use them fresh to make a tincture. Use for nervous tension and insomnia, for lack of appetite, sluggish digestion and as a liver tonic.

Drying Herbs, page 42
Making Tinctures, page 46

HOP BEER

> 4.6 litres (1 gallon) boiling water
> 15g (½oz) dried hop flowers
> 450g (1lb) malt extract
> 450g (1lb) light brown sugar
> 1 tablespoon dried yeast
> Extra 4 tablespoons brown sugar for bottling

Method

1. Boil the hops in the water for about an hour.

2. Strain off the hops through muslin into a clean bucket, and top back up to 4.6 litres (1 gallon) again with cooled boiled water.

3. When lukewarm, sprinkle yeast over the top, cover with a lid or clean tea towel, wrapped round with string.

4. Leave for three days or so until fermentation has finished.

5. Rack off the beer and bottle, adding ½ teaspoon of sugar to each bottle and seal tightly.

6. Open in about a week when the sediment has settled.

Rowan berries were also traditionally brewed into ale in Wales, and heather ale is made in Scotland. Worth experimenting with by using the above recipe.

Making Dark Storage Jars

All herbal preparations from tinctures to syrups and vinegars are best stored in dark jars or bottles as light destroys their herbal properties. If your herbs are kept in a dark cupboard it is fine to use clear jars. If they are kept out then the jars need to be made dark by any of the following methods.

1. Clear jars can be painted with dark glass paints. They can also be painted with acrylics or blackboard paint with designs added on top once it is dry.

2. Wrap dark cloth around them. T-shirt material is best because it stretches and is a great use of old T-shirts. Cut long strips of material and wrap round the jar. Wind the wool around in random or neat patterns. These can look really beautiful. Alternatively wrap the jar in dark wools.

3. Glue dark tissue paper onto the jar. Pressed flowers or leaves can also be added. Once the glue is dry, paint with varnish.

4. Put the clear glass jar in a clean or new black sock and tie it round with coloured thread.

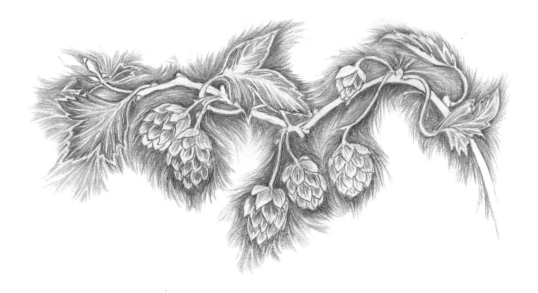

SEASONAL CELEBRATIONS

❀ Lammas or Lughnasadh

❀ Finding and Crafting Your Own Staff or Walking Stick

❀ Making Smudge Sticks

This is the beginning of the harvest time when the sun and the rains swell the seeds and ripen the fruits. Misty mornings and colder nights remind us that we have passed the longest day, and the cycle of the year is turning, as we dance on the edge between high summer and the edge of autumn.

This is the time of high days and holidays and a celebration of the abundance and richness of our lives and the Earth. People are out and about, making things happen, visiting friends and family, exploring, going on holiday, going to festivals and community gatherings, making new friends, falling in love, falling out of love, walking the land, swimming in rivers, lakes and the sea.

It is a time when we can feel most alive, full of hope, rich with connection, friendships and community. But we can also feel lonely and vulnerable. This is a call to be honest and real about our feelings and not to stay isolated by them.

Sharing our feelings helps others to share theirs. It is a gift we give each other. Expressing our feelings helps us to flow and to see what we want to change and what we still need to work with. They are the new seeds of our future selves forming.

Lammas or Lughnasadh
End of July – Beginning of August

Traditionally Lammas is a celebration of the great gathering in of the grain harvest, stored throughout the winter to keep us in bread and grain products. They are also the seeds that will be sown in the spring and the seeds that will bring next year's harvest.

This is a time for community gatherings, fairs, camps and festivals. In the past, the great Lammas fairs would last a month, and provide, much as our gatherings do today, an opportunity for people to share their harvest of achievements, their wares and produce, music, theatre, ideas, and to celebrate the abundance of the summer.

Lammas encourages our generosity of spirit and reminds us to give thanks for all the abundance in our lives. The more we give from our hearts, the more returns to us – as all is connected and flowing parts of the whole.

Much is coming to fruition now as the season of active outer growth is coming to an end and the season of inner reflection begins.

Lammas Celebrations
Included here are some ideas for connecting to the Earth, the seasonal energy, and your inner wisdom. Choose a couple of things to do, and be open to your own spontaneous inspirations of the moment.

For insights and overview about co-creating seasonal gatherings, see page 66

• At the full moon, invite friends of all generations for an evening picnic, and ask everyone to bring drums and percussion, musical instruments, a song, a play or a poem to recite. Bring seasonal food and drinks for a feast and some wood for a fire. Stay up late around an outdoor fire, fire gaze and share stories and entertain each other. Look for shooting stars and make a wish.

- Ask everyone to bring something for a 'Basket Of Abundance'. Put something in, take something out and give thanks for your abundance.

- Ask everyone to bring home made bread, cakes and biscuits made from different grain flours and other seasonal food to share. Lay these on a colourful cloth and create a beautiful shrine of abundance with the food at the centre. Decorate with grasses and wild flowers.

- Make simple head-dresses from twisted and bound grasses and wild flowers. The sticky long stalks of cleavers make instant circlets that can be used as a basis for further weavings.

- Make simple 'corn dolls' or 'harvest dolls' by the same method. Weave in your thanks for your own abundance and the abundance of the Earth.

- Ask everyone to bring ribbons to share and have a basket ready where people can put them and a pair of scissors. Each ribbon represents your thanks for an aspect of your life that is coming to fruition, a celebration and thanksgiving of your abundance, or an aspect of the Earth you love and pledge to help. The ribbons are tied with due ceremony to your headdress, round your wrist, in your hair or hung in the trees.

Alternatively, everyone sits in a circle and the basket of ribbons are passed round. Each take three ribbons and then take it in turn to share with each other three things you celebrate at this time. Encourage each other to celebrate their achievements both outer and inner, to celebrate our beautiful Earth and to make a pledge to help her.

- Pass round a wooden bowl or pouch of organic wholewheat grains. Each take a few grains and hold them while meditating on your achievements this year. Traditionally this is a time of assessment so ask yourself how the season of growth has gone for you. Seek the seeds hidden within your personal harvest that you will take into the autumn and winter.

- Ask everyone to bring homemade bread, a bottle of spring water and a glass. Put them all in the centre of the circle. Spend some time in thanks and reflective meditation, giving thanks for our abundance of bread and water and an awareness of those who are hungry and thirsty in the world.

Tear up some of the bread into a basket and pass it around the circle. Each takes a piece of bread, give thanks for their abundance and shares any thoughts on how we might help others to have more.

Fill your glass with spring water and hold it to your heart. Spend some time in meditation and see what messages you receive. Send a prayer of thanks to the water. Call out a toast to energise a vision of a world wide commitment to clean water for everyone. Follow with other toasts in celebration of water.

• Changing Our Conversation: Our survival as a species depends on our being adaptable, able to move out of old habits and be open to new ways forward. Celebrate what is on the move for you. What new things have grown in you this summer? What do you choose to change? What lifestyle changes will you begin now? What other ways will help you to adapt to the changes coming? Look for new phrases you can say that will help you to move more fully towards a holistic perspective and a joy of change. Share these reflections with each other or write in your journal.

• Make an Earth Necklace: Ask everyone to bring natural beads to share. Dedicate each bead as you thread it to an aspect of Earth awareness you wish to strengthen, and to new ways forward you wish to take. Each bead strengthens your awareness of your special contribution and the part you have to play in helping the Earth to repair. Encourage everyone to work in contemplative silence. If indoors, play some music to help this.

Intuit an Earth-tribe name for yourself and take it in turns to name each other as the necklace is placed over the head.

• Earth Offering Ceremony: Ask everyone to bring flowers, petals, seeds and grain as an offering to the Earth. Have a beautiful wooden bowl at the centre of the circle and invite each person to sit in the circle around it and speak about their love for the Earth and about the things they have bought for their offering. They then add their offering to the central bowl. When everyone has had their say, someone carries the bowl outside to a significant spot and all follow in silence or toning, humming or singing a chant. Each person takes a handful of the offering and gives it to the Earth with their love and a pledge to be part of her human support system and to live life with care and awareness of the Earth's needs.

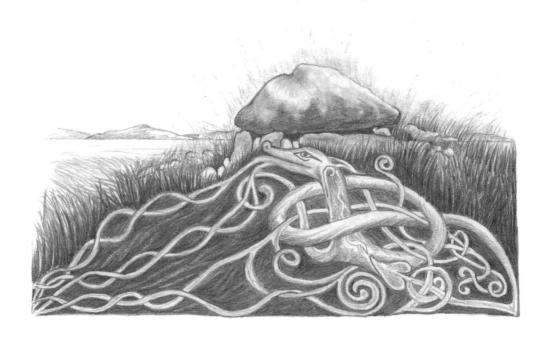

Finding and Crafting Your Own Staff or Walking Stick

There is something profoundly bonding about finding, cutting and crafting your own staff or walking stick from a location you can return to in your mind's eye.

1. While out walking keep an eye open for straight lengths of stick that might be suitable. Occasionally you can find a stick that is the right size and has a natural spiral up the shaft created by honeysuckle. Hazel is the obvious choice as they naturally send up many straight sticks from the base of their trunks. These are not the nut bearing branches and the more you cut them, the more will grow. Straight sticks can also be found on hawthorn, birch, rowan, holly, willow, ash and blackthorn. (Be careful of the blackthorn spikes as scratches can turn septic.) All of these native trees coppice well and if you have space to grow trees, do some coppicing of your own to encourage new straight growth for staffs and walking sticks. Each tree species has its own energy and gifts. Intuit what they are for you.

Making a Talking Stick, page 240

2. Other considerations to bear in mind are the weight, the thickness of the shaft, the height you need and the type of handle (if any) you want and whether it would be alright to cut the stick – depending on where it is growing.

3. When you think you have found the right piece of wood, in a location that would be suitable to cut from, next you have to ask the tree for permission. Unless you get a recoil or an uneasy feeling then it is probably fine to cut it. Only you will know. Give thanks before and after cutting, and rub the stump with moss and soil. Have a few minutes with the tree while the shock settles.

4. Strip off any side branches and get the height right while you are in situ and walk away bonding with your new staff or stick.

5. If you want to take the bark off, do it within hours of cutting the stick. In many cases it will peel right off in long strips that follow the natural contours of the wood. Leave the stripped wood somewhere it can dry out gradually, like in an outhouse or garage. If you leave it outside the wood will go grey. Bark can also be stripped off later with a penknife, but the stick will need to be sanded down to get rid of all the blade marks.

6. Any carving is also initially done within a few weeks while the wood is still soft and green, although you do have to be careful after carving green wood to let the wood dry out slowly as it can split. Decide on how you want the top, shaping it with a knife and creating something that is comfortable to hold. As the wood dries out use a rough sandpaper to take off the main blade marks and ever-finer sandpapers to bring the wood up to a smooth finish. Every tree has a different coloured wood, a different feel, a different way of working, with varying hardness and density.

7. If you decide to leave the bark on then let the stick dry out naturally in the wind and the rain or in an out house or porch. You can still use it for walks. Leave it natural or once the bark is completely dry you can gently rub with a fine sandpaper to bring out the patterns of the bark, and smooth off any rough bits.

8. When the stick is dry, oil it to keep the wood fed and to bring out the colours. I use any of the macerated herbal oils I have made, adding another layer of energy to the stick.

Making Smudge Sticks

Smudging is a traditional way of cleansing and clearing energy. A bundle of dried herbs is lit and blown out and the glowing embers are blown on so that it smoulders and smokes. The smoke is then wafted around a space or person for cleansing or to clear away any stuck or negative energy. They can be made of mixed bundles of herbs or a single herb.

MUGWORT (*Artemisia vulgaris*) and **WORMWOOD** (*Artemisia absinthium*)
Native plants that have a long tradition of being used for burning, bringing clarity and insight.

COLTSFOOT (*Tussilago farfara*) and **MULLEIN** (*Verbascum thapsus*)
Both burn well and give off a smoke that is beneficial to the lungs.

SAGE, ROSEMARY, THYME
All are aromatic kitchen garden herbs that have a lot of oil in their leaves and will burn well and smell good.

Any of the pines or cedars burn well for the same reason.

Method

1. Cut the herbs the day before you need them. They will wilt overnight and be much easier to bind together the next day.

2. Tie the stems together using natural material such as hemp string, cotton or raffia. Leave two long lengths of thread.

3. Using one of the threads wrap the bundle of herbs as tightly as you can as you winding down to the bottom of the bundle and back up again. Tie it off at the top and then do the same with the other length and tie it off again. Make a hanging loop.

4. Hang in a warm dry place to completely dry out before use.

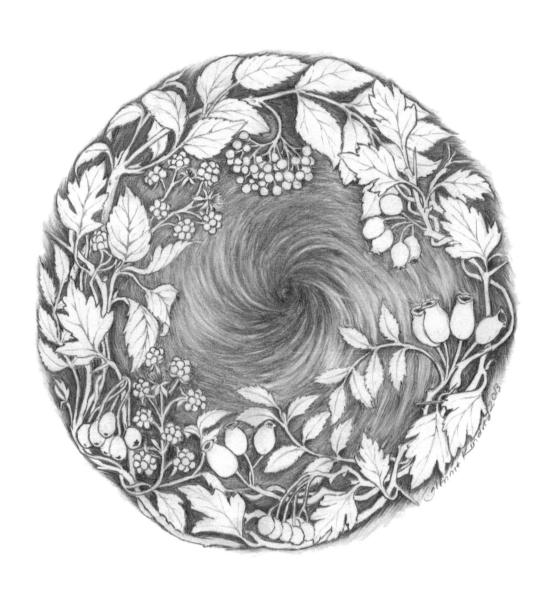

AUTUMN'S
wild edge

September into October

The Earth's energy is settling, the outer growth cycle is finishing and it will soon be time for the Earth and us, to rest again. There is a shift in the weather, a wildness blows in on colder winds and there is a sense that summer is over. We begin to feel the pull to prepare for the winter months as new possibilities begin to reveal themselves.

The life force goes into swelling the fruit and the seeds within the fruits. It is a time of nature's wild abundance and a natural time to give thanks for all the abundance the Earth has given us this year. We give thanks for our personal harvest, our friendships, the adventures we have had, all that we have loved and appreciated, honouring our losses too as part of the whole.

OUT ON THE LAND

❀ Natural Darkness ❀ Inspiration from Nature
❀ Collecting Native Tree Seeds
❀ Making a Foraging Stick
❀ Foraging for Fruit and Mushrooms

It is time for wild blustery walks on the land, picking fruit from the wild edges of the fields and lanes. At this time of year never set out without plastic tubs for blackberries and elderberries, paper bags for sloes, rosehips, haws, seeds, nuts, wild apples and wild plums. At this time of year there are always new treasures to gather, and finding edible mushrooms is always a treat. Remember to step outside often to keep your connection to the land, especially when the day is dark. It is always much lighter outside and once out in the elements a fresh vigour and happiness fills you.

This is the time of the Autumn Equinox, when day and night are equal length, and light and dark are in balance. As you walk reflect on where you feel you have achieved a greater balance this year. What areas of your life do you feel are still out of balance? What do you feel you need to change in order to encourage more balance?

It is time for inner change as we go into the dark cycle and we assimilate and learn from our experiences of the summer. Like the plants and trees, we can shed the old leaves of our year's outer growth and send the roots of our future happiness down deeper into the dark fertility within us. This strengthens us from the inside and brings us lasting stability.

Natural Darkness

Many of us have become afraid to be out in nature in the dark. By turning to face this fear we empower ourselves once again to become comfortable with all aspects of our whole selves. Practise first by stepping out into the garden. Chances are with all the streetlights it will not be very dark, but it's a start. Look for any dark pockets you might explore. Expand your senses, especially your hearing, and listen out for the calls of the night creatures.

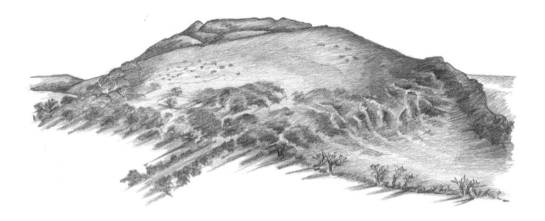

If you have dark country lanes nearby try walking in them with a friend. Walk in silence and walk as quietly as you can. See how your eyes become attuned to the dark and your sense of hearing sharpens. What calls can you hear? Learn to recognise them and practise imitating them. You may be rewarded by seeing glow worms or fireflies.

Bats, cats, foxes, badgers, hedgehogs, deer, otters and owls all live on the edge between twilight and the dark. Many birds migrate in the dark and navigate by the stars. At night in the autumn you can hear their calls as they keep in contact with each other on their epic voyages.

Choose not to be disabled by the dark, but enabled by a new confidence, with a greater awareness and honing of each of your five outer senses. Decide to develop your inner senses, your intuitive abilities and your natural instincts.

Inspiration From Nature

Earth-based cultures believe that the natural world is alive with significance and spirit teachings. Seeing, hearing or encountering animals, birds, reptiles or insects when out walking on the land, or in a dream or waking vision, would be seen as the spirit-world sending you a teaching. Your understanding of that creature, its habits and habitat are all part of how you intuit the teaching and its relevance to you in the moment.

You can wait for this to happen naturally or see what is revealed to you via a simple exercise: Settle yourself into the landscape, perhaps with a tree, or by water.

Feel your breathing become steady as you find your sense of oneness and peace with the natural world around you. Bring a question into your heart, something you need guidance with. Close your eyes and stay focused on the question. When you feel ready open your eyes and see what your gaze rests on. What you see is an inspiration from nature's wisdom, a message. Your interpretation unlocks the understanding and helps reveal your own inner wisdom.

Collecting Native Tree Seeds

Acorns, Haws, Alder cones, Hazel nuts, Holly berries, Elder berries

There is something so profound about a tiny tree seed and its potential to grow into a beautiful large tree. A tree will produce hundreds of seeds, but often there is little room for them to spread naturally. And yet we need more trees in our environment. We can all help by taking some of their bountiful seed harvest each year to grow and nurture a few tree seeds until they grow into large enough trees to plant out.

Look for seeds from the healthiest and strongest trees. It is always best to collect seeds from the native trees growing in your own area. They have adapted to the local climate and soil as well as the insects that live there. Pick the seeds directly from the tree or when they are newly fallen. Don't collect the first seeds that fall as the later ones will be better quality. Only take what you know you will use as these nuts and fruits are food for the birds and wildlife. Put the seeds in labelled paper bags.

When you get home, sort through them and pick out the best ones for growing. Return the rest to the Earth with your thanks. Tree seeds are best planted straight away without letting them dry out. Sprinkle them into labelled pots of compost or compost and sharp sand or in labelled holding beds and water well. If there is danger of rodents digging them up, cover with fine mesh. They should sprout in the spring, although some take two years.

Making a Foraging Stick

While watching a programme about aboriginal women foraging in the bush, I noticed they each had a special foraging stick with a hook at one end and a sharp point at the other. Perhaps this useful tool was used by our own hunter-gatherer ancestors? The hook is used for hooking down branches when gathering wild fruit and the pointed end is used for digging. I immediately began looking for a suitable piece of wood to cut.

Obviously the size of this tool is up to you but my recommendation is for it to feel comfortable in your hand, to be of a good weight for you to enjoy using, and the length of it will slip down the side of your day bag or rucksack.

The shape of the hook is important and this takes time to find. It also preferably needs to be made from a hard wood such as hawthorn, oak, holly or apple.

Once you have found your piece of wood and cut it with due respect and thanks, cut off any rough bits and whittle them smooth, and sharpen the stick end. Later when your foraging stick has dried out, you can sand any rough edges and give the whole thing an oiling to stop the wood from drying out.

Foraging For Fruit and Mushrooms

The fruits are ripening now and many a snack can be had while out walking the land. Make sure the area feels safe to eat from and don't eat or collect if the bushes look damaged or the leaves look brown and withered, even if the fruit looks fine.

At this time of year never leave home without collecting bags, plastic tubs for soft fruit, and your foraging stick if you have made one!

Traditionally some fruit is always left on a tree and the tree is thanked. Pick with sensitivity and remember to leave plenty of everything for the birds and wildlife as this is their winter food we are picking.

It is also mushroom season, and although this book does not cover mushrooms and fungi, these opportunities for the wild food forager are not to be missed. There are some easily identifiable mushrooms in this country that are safe to eat and not confused with anything toxic. So get a good field guide and learn what they are, how to be sure of identifying them and how to pick them correctly.

Foraging, page 17

THE WILD GARDENER

❀ A Balanced Approach to Autumn ❀ Seed Collecting
❀ Sowing Native Winter Greens
❀ Transplanting and Dividing Roots
❀ Planting Native Bulbs ❀ The Productive Lawn
❀ Guerrilla Gardening – Native Bulbs

Autumn can be a busy time in the garden with the days shortening, winter approaching and fruit to pick and store. It's always a joy to see everything gathered in and to celebrate nature's abundant harvest. Autumn is the beginning of root energy when plants can be divided and transplanted, trees can be moved or planted out and bulbs are planted.

As the colours change and leaves fall we too begin to respond to the change in the weather and prepare for a new set of conditions that the winter months will bring.

A Balanced Approach to Autumn

There are two approaches for the wild gardener at this time of year. One option is to do very little in the garden, let the plants die back naturally and compost the soil with their own leaves. This leaves seed heads for the seed eating birds and leaves the ground undisturbed for the wildlife to find where it wants to burrow into and hibernate. Everything eventually dies back and composts of its own accord without our intervention.

Some plants and bushes will benefit from being cut back. It helps hedges to thicken and stops garden trees from getting too big. When the buds begin to form during the winter, they will then be putting their energy into next year's growth. Tree and hedge trimmings can be piled along the edges of the garden for wildlife to hibernate in.

I take a balanced approach to autumn and walk the middle way. I tidy up parts of the garden, shutting down some of the empty growing beds for next year by spreading them with a layer of manure and compost mix. All the little creatures that live in the soil pull it all down during the winter and it improves the life and energy of the soil ready for planting in the spring. I let the edges stay wild, leaving plenty for the birds to eat and creating plenty of places to encourage safe hibernation for all the wildlife I love to share this garden with.

Seed Collecting

Many seeds will be falling and sowing themselves now but if you want to collect them and sow them in the spring yourself, then choose dry sunny days to gather any seeds that fall when shaken into dishes or brown paper bags. Sort through what you have picked, taking out the best ones and put them in clean labelled brown paper bags to dry out some where warm. Return the rest to the wild edges for birds and other creatures to find or maybe to grow.

Shake the seed bags frequently until you are satisfied they are properly dried and then transfer the seeds to old envelopes. Label them and add any growing tips you have learnt about the plants and store in your seed box in a cool dry place.

Leave some seeds on the plants to self-seed in their own wild way. Any self-seeded seedlings can be dug up in the spring, planted out or potted up and passed on to friends.

Sowing Native Winter Greens

Cleavers, Corn Salad, Salad Burnet, Winter Cress

It seems crazy to be sowing seeds at this time of year, but this ensures edible greens you can pick in the winter and early spring. You need to get the seeds in by early September so the plants can get started while the weather is still warm. Some can be sprinkled directly in the ground, others benefit from being sown and planted out in a cloche or in tubs up by the house where you can keep an eye on them.

CLEAVERS
Pick the sticky seeds and sprinkle them in large pots for an early spring crop. If cleavers is treated like a crop and picked frequently, then an endless supply of the delicious tips keep growing. The plant is contained and doesn't get the chance to ramble all over the garden.

225

CORN SALAD

If you haven't a dedicated bed for self-seeded plants then sow the seeds now for early spring crops. They can be sprinkled in cloches for added protection or in any bed that remains largely undisturbed from now on and will catch the winter sun.

SALAD BURNET

Sow these in pots for an early salad crop next spring. They keep growing throughout the winter. The more you pick, the more fresh leaves appear. Don't put them in the cloche as they don't need it and take up too much room in the spring.

WINTER CRESS

Sow now for plenty of fresh winter and spring leaves.

Transplanting and Dividing Roots

Lady's Smock, Lady's Mantle, Sorrel, Yarrow

All of these native plants can be eaten in the winter and early spring so it is worth encouraging them by transplanting and dividing large clumps to make new plants. These can be moved around the garden to more appropriate places, potted up for guerrilla gardening activities or given to friends.

Yarrow is particularly useful around the garden as it is beneficial to any plant it grows alongside and will increase the yields and flavour of other herbs.

Plant Reference Guide, page 249

Planting Native Bulbs

Planting bulbs that will come up in the spring is a great pleasure of autumn gardening. Many native bulbs have all but disappeared from the wild, but they are suited to our damp climate and once established should thrive. There are many beautiful native bulbs worth growing in the garden and as always if you want to plant bulbs in the wild, only plant native ones.

N.B. Most of the following plants are NOT EDIBLE and some are poisonous.

BABINGTON'S LEEK (*Allium babingtonii*)

A native bulb which grows to 2m (6½ft) high. Looks good *en masse* in a border. Rare in the wild but sometimes found growing in rocky clefts and sandy places along the coasts of Cornwall, Dorset and West Ireland. Flowers July to August.

BLUEBELL OR WILD HYACINTH (*Endymion non-scriptus*)

A native of woodlands, they grow best in undisturbed soil and will grow in the shade. It is a protected plant in the wild although they are not considered to be under immediate threat. The biggest concern is the cross-pollination with numerous hybrids and imported species such as the more robust Spanish Bluebell (*H. hispanica*). It is important that we plant the native variety, especially when considering planting them out. Highly poisonous. Flowers April to June.

CHIVES (*Allium schoenoprasum*)

The flowers of this native bulb look wonderful in the flowerbed, and you can eat them too. Considered to be a 'nurse' plant, this will help any plant it is planted alongside. They can be grown from seed or large clumps can be split in the autumn. They prefer full sun. Flowers June to July.

LODDON LILY OR SUMMER SNOWFLAKE (*Leucojum aestivum*)

Protected in the wild this native bulb grows along riverbanks, in damp soil beneath alders and willows, and in damp meadows and woodland. The beautiful white flowers with green tips grow to about 46cm (18in) high and resemble a snowdrop in appearance. Flowers April to May.

ROUND-HEADED LEEK (*Allium sphaerocephalon*)

Similar to the Babington's leek, rare in the wild now. Flowers June to August.

SNAKE'S HEAD FRITILLARY (*Fritillaria meleagris*)

Occurs naturally in damp meadows in southern England but now rare in the wild. Handle the delicate bulbs carefully when planting out and plant them 10cm (4in) deep. They like damp conditions but full sun. Absolutely fine to plant under turf as this was once a plant of grasslands. Flowers April to May.

SNOW DROP (*Galanthus nivalis*)

Native of Wales and the West, found in damp valleys, in woods and along streams. Flowers January to March.

Star of Bethlehem (*Ornithogalum umbellatum*)
Native only in the East of England but found all over northern Europe and was once eaten as a survival food by those on pilgrimage to the Holy Land. It will grow on most soils and prefers to grow through grass. Flowers April – May.

Wild Leek (*Allium ampeloprasum*)
A native bulb, now rare in the wild but can be found growing along the coast in Cornwall, Somerset and South Wales. Flowers July to August.

Wild Daffodil (*Narcissus pseudonarcissus*)
The native daffodil has a small pale head, and once filled our damp meadows and woodlands in the spring. Flowers February to April.

Most native bulbs will push up through grass. Lift the turf in the autumn, loosen the soil, plant them and put the turf back. They will grow through the grass in the spring.

Native Plant, Seed and Bulb Suppliers, page 283

The Productive Lawn

Time to rethink lawns. Lets face it, they need a lot of upkeep and for me, in their present format, they have had their day.

Gradually over the last few years I have been adding different plants to my lawn and slowly it is becoming a bit of a wild flower meadow and is very beautiful at different times of the year. A quick mow or trim with the shears gives it a little spruce up twice a year in early summer after the first flush of spring flowers and about this time in autumn. The rest of the time it looks stunning covered with wild flowers, some of which can be harvested for food, and some for medicines.

Give the lawn its autumn tidy-up and then transplant plants or scatter the seeds of meadow or grassland native plants into the lawn. The lawn then becomes a productive resource for edible plants and medicines.

Betony (*Stachys officinalis*)
A native perennial and an attractive garden plant with many medicinal uses.

Plant Reference Guide, page 250

COMMON SPEEDWELL (*Veronica officinalis*)

A native perennial of heaths and grasslands. Another important medicinal herb of the past, once used for bronchitis, whooping cough, indigestion, gout, bladder stones, rheumatism and liver complaints.

EYEBRIGHT (*Euphrasia officinalis*)

A native annual of grasslands that grows with and in grass. Use an infusion of the leaves to bathe sore, tired, watery and sensitive eyes and for conjunctivitis. It is a good tonic and cleanser that has a beneficial effect on the whole system, clearing out toxins and mucus and improving a sluggish liver. Use as a gargle for sore throats and catarrh and for earache.

HEARTSEASE (*Viola tricolor*)

A native annual of grasslands, wastelands, fields and gardens, also known as Wild Pansy. The flowers can be eaten in salads.

LADY'S SMOCK (*Cardamine pratensis*)

A native perennial found in damp meadows. The leaves can be eaten throughout the year and are rich in vitamin C.

Plant Reference Guide, page 265

RED CLOVER (*Trifolium pratense*)

A native perennial found growing in grass. A nitrogen-fixer that will enrich the soil and a prized herbal remedy.

Plant Reference Guide, page 269

SALAD BURNET (*Sanguisorba minor*)

A native perennial found in meadows and dry pastures. Eat the leaves throughout the year until it flowers, May to August.

SELF HEAL (*Prunella vulgaris*)

A native perennial and attractive garden plant with bright purple flowers, much loved by the bees. An important immune system herb.

Plant Reference Guide, page 273

SORREL (*Rumex acestosa*)

A native perennial found in grassland, in pastures and along roadsides.

The small arrow shaped leaves taste good in salads and spinach mixes.

Plant Reference Guide, page 274

YARROW (*Achillea millefolium*)
A common native perennial with edible leaves and many medicinal uses.

Plant Reference Guide, page 280

Guerrilla Gardening – Native Bulbs

Native bulbs can be quickly planted out by the guerrilla gardener, using a sharp bulb trowel. They will remain hidden until the spring when their appearance will lift the spirits and bring delight. As many of them originated in woodland, they are ideal for shady and forgotten corners. Plant them under trees, by springs and wells and along the edges of walls and footpaths. They will happily grow through grass so gently lift the turf, dig a hole and pop them in, putting the turf back with as little disturbance as possible. If they remain undisturbed for many years they will spread.

Native Plant, Seed and Bulb Suppliers, page 283

KITCHEN MEDICINE

❀ Drying Berries and Fruit

❀ Fruit Tinctures and Elixirs – Elderberry Elixir

❀ Fruit Syrups ❀ Fruit Honeys

❀ Fruit Wines ❀ Fruit Brandy

❀ Fruit Jam and Jelly ❀ Fruit Chutney

Collecting fruit is a prime pastime at this time of the year, whether it is foraging along the hedgerows, in the garden, or from locations found around the town. This is the season for making berry tinctures and honey elixirs to boost the immune system and potions to gladden the heart in the depths of darkest winter. Make the most of the fruit by making wines, ciders, fruit spirits, vinegars, jams, chutneys and pickles and not forgetting fruit pies and crumbles!

Drying Berries and Fruit

Elderberries, Haws, Rosehips, Rowan berries

As always collect on a dry day, thanking the tree for its gifts. Bring home and sort through, discarding any that are blemished or soft. Lay them out between two paper sheets somewhere warm and dry, and out of direct sunlight. When they have begun to dry out, transfer into clean brown paper bags and put on top of the radiators, near the cooker, or wood-burner and shake every day or two.

When they are completely dry, store them in labelled dark glass jars or brown paper bags. When you need them, make a decoction by soaking the berries overnight in cold water.

N.B. The seeds of rosehips are an irritant and must not be internalised. Deseed them while they are fresh. Cut them open and scoop out the seeds. Wash well and spread out to dry, turning frequently.

Decoctions, page 231
Plant Reference Guide, page 249

Fruit Tinctures and Elixirs

Elder berries, Haws and Rosehips

Check the properties of the above fruits and make plenty of these fruit tinctures and elixirs for the winter medicine cupboard.

N.B. For adults only because of alcohol content.

Plant Reference Guide, page 249
Making Tinctures, page 46
Making Elixirs, page 48

ELDERBERRY ELIXIR

It is worth making lots of this excellent immune system booster and having plenty to give away to family and friends.

1. Half fill a jar with elderberries, add star anise, cloves and cinnamon bark and half fill with honey.

2. Prod and mix well with a chop stick to remove the air bubbles and then top up with brandy. Stir well.

3. Shake every few days for a month and then strain and rebottle into dropper bottles.

4. Take neat or add to water, hot or cold. This is a truly delicious way to take your medicine!

Fruit Syrups

Rosehips, Hawthorn, Blackberry, Elderberry

Any fruit can be made into a fruit syrup, which are good for children.

For the method, see Making Herbal Syrups, page 163

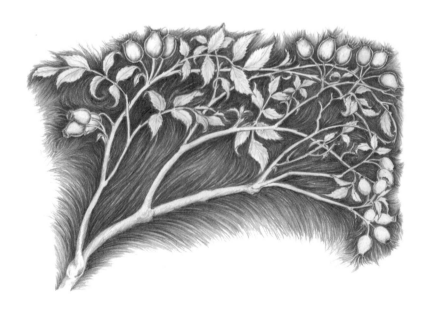

Elderberry Syrup

This is different from the other syrups as it has additional spices added. Highly prized and praised, and well worth making! It does the same job as the tincture but without the alcohol, so it is good for children. Elderberry syrup is wonderful for chesty coughs and sore throats. It boosts the immune system and when taken at the first sign of a cold can prevent it from happening altogether!

Method

1. Strip elderberries into a large pan. Add a cinnamon stick (broken up), chopped lemons, a few star anise, cloves, all spice, some slices of ginger… Be intuitive with these! Stir it up and let the mixture stand overnight.

2. The next day warm gently on a really low heat, bringing it up to boiling, and letting the juices flow.

3. When cool, strain through muslin or a clean cotton pillowcase, squeezing all the juices out.

4. Measure the liquid. You will need the same amount of clear honey to liquid.

5. Return to a clean pan. Heat gently and when hot but not boiling, stir in the honey and when it has completely dissolved, pour into sterilised dark bottles. Tighten the lids while hot. Label and date.

6. Take by the teaspoonful or drink as a warming and healing cordial by adding hot water. Once opened it needs to be kept in the fridge and will last a few weeks. Unopened it will last for a year until you are ready to make your next batch!

The dose is a teaspoonful at a time, taken frequently.
N.B. Halve the amount for children. Do not give to children under 3.

Fruit Honeys

Elderberry, Blackberry, Rosehips (deseeded)

Well worth making to enjoy during the winter months. Make them into drinks or pour over yogurt or ice cream and to zing up other puddings.

Making Herbal Honeys, page 51

233

Fruit Wines

Crab Apple, Blackberry, Haw, Elderberry, Rosehips (deseeded)

All edible fruit makes good wine and the addition of extra spices, or combinations of fruit makes for interesting creations.

Fruit Wines, page 207

ELDERBERRY WINE
This is a rich dark wine that never fails! Take hot before bed to bring out a cold or fever.

Ingredients
4.5 litres (8 pint) glasses of elderberries
4 litres (7 pints) of water
14g (½oz) chopped root ginger
7g (¼oz) of cloves
1 teaspoon yeast
900g (2lb) sugar

Method
1. De-stalk the berries and put in a plastic bucket with 4 litres of boiling water.

2. Leave for 3 days, stirring every day so that no mould develops.

3. Strain off the fruit into a jam pan, and add the finely chopped ginger and cloves and bring slowly almost up to the boil. Turn off the heat.

4. Add the sugar and stir to dissolve and return to the clean bucket, straining off the cloves and ginger.

5. Let it cool to lukewarm and stir in the yeast.

6. Pour into a demijohn, fit the fermentation lock and leave until it stops fermenting.

7. Carefully siphon off into clean dark wine bottles, label and date.

   Keep for 2 years if possible before drinking.

Fruit Brandy

Elderberry Brandy, Haw Brandy, Rosehip Brandy, Rowan Berry Brandy

Edible native fruits can be preserved in brandy, with sugar. Their flavour and herbal properties are released into the spirit and create a delicious liqueur.

Method
1. Find a dark jar or wide-necked bottle (Allow for the fact that the fruit will swell slightly) and nearly fill with the best and cleanest fruit.

2. Cover with sugar and fill the jar up with brandy.

3. Shake gently every few days for 6 weeks or so.

4. Strain off the fruit and re-bottle in time for Christmas, although it improves with age.

Fruit Jam and Jelly

Homemade wild fruit jam is a treat for the winter.

CRAB APPLE JELLY
1. Rough chop 2.7kg (6lb) of fruit and boil in water with a slice of ginger root and a chopped lemon.

2. Pour the pulp into a jelly bag and let it drip overnight. Do not squeeze!

3. Return the liquid to the pan and add a pound of sugar to each pint of juice. Rapid boil for 15 minutes or so, until the jelly shows signs of setting when tested on a cold plate.

4. Pour into hot jam jars that have been sterilized for 10 minutes in a hot oven.

ROWAN BERRY JELLY
The addition of crab apples with the rowan berries means this is not a clear jelly but the taste is milder and more palatable. Good on bread, porridge and ice cream. Use only rowan berries if you want the traditional sharp rowan berry jelly, which is similar to cranberry jelly and eaten with savoury dishes.

Method

1. In 1 litre (2 pints) of water, boil 900g (2lb) of rough chopped crab apples and 1.35kg (3lb) rowan berries stripped from their stalks, until it becomes a pulp.

2. Follow steps 2–4 for Crab Apple Jelly above.

ELDERBERRY AND APPLE JAM

This has a great flavour and is quick and easy to make.

1. Make a pulp by boiling 900g (2lb) of roughly chopped apples (use windfalls) in some water, and pass through a sieve to remove the cores, skins and seeds.

2. Do the same with 900g (2lb) of elderberries, removed from the stalks, with a little water as they are so juicy, and sieve to remove the seeds and skins.

3. Combine the two liquids and measure.

4. Return to a clean pan and add 450g (1lb) of sugar per pint of liquid. Stir well.

5. Bring back to the boil. Boil for around 10 minutes until it shows signs of thickening. Pour into hot sterilised jars. Put the lids on straight away and tighten.

6. Then when cool tighten the lids again, label and date.

Fruit Chutneys

APPLE AND ELDERBERRY CHUTNEY

Experiment using this basic recipe for chutney:

Ingredients
900g (2lb) of elderberries (removed from the stalks)
450g (1lb) apples (peeled, cored and chopped)
A handful of sultanas
1 large chopped onion
1 pint of vinegar
3 tablespoons sugar
Salt and pepper to taste

Method

1. In a large pan combine the ingredients:

2. Add 1 teaspoon each of salt, crushed peppercorns, chopped ginger, crushed mustard seeds and mixed spice.

3. Bring to the boil and simmer until it thickens. Test the flavour and adjust to taste with more or less salt, pepper or sugar.

4. Pour into jars that have been sterilised in a hot oven and screw on lids.

5. Tighten the lids again when cold, label and date.

SEASONAL CELEBRATIONS

❀ Autumn Equinox
❀ Making a Talking Stick ❀ Making your own Incense

This is a time of harvest and thanksgiving, a celebration of the Earth's great abundance and our own. As we appreciate the beauty of the Earth and her bountiful harvest, we also look at our own personal harvest, celebrate what has come to fruition this year, and count each and every blessing in our lives. We take this energy of appreciation inside ourselves as we turn to welcome and value the gifts that the new inner cycle will bring.

Autumn Equinox
20th – 23rd September

Once again day and night, light and dark, are equal, reminding us to find the balanced edge of equilibrium between our outer and inner selves.

Autumn Equinox marks the final end of the outer growth cycle. It is a time of change, with high tides, wild changeable weather and wild uncertainties as we plan what to do next. The shorter colder days and colder longer nights affect these decisions. We recognise this as a transition point, an opportunity for a new set of possibilities and the opportunity to grow in new ways. We take all we have learnt during the spring and summer and transform them by taking them within us.

We walk the outer ways and walk the inner ways, and aim to flow in poise and balance in the wild edges in between.

AUTUMN EQUINOX CELEBRATIONS

Included here are some ideas for connecting to the Earth, the seasonal energy, and your inner wisdom. Choose a couple of things to do, and be open to your own spontaneous inspirations of the moment.

For insights and overview about co-creating seasonal gatherings, see page 66

• Welcome in the changing season and the Autumn Equinox with a day out walking the land. Either plan to go on the actual day whatever the weather, or decide spontaneously when a fine wild Equinox day presents itself. Make a pilgrimage to a special place or plan a vision quest or retreat. Review the last 6 months since the Spring Equinox and seek answers for what you plan to do next as winter approaches. Walk barefoot where you can and seek help from the wisdom of the Earth and her teachings. Explore the wild edges of your intuition and magical self. Be open to your spontaneity and your own true inner wisdom.

Vision Quest, page 15

• Invite friends for an evening round an outdoor fire. Ask everyone to bring seasonal food and drinks to share and have a table ready to put these on. If the weather takes you indoors then fill a large bowl with earth or sand and fill with candles to create an 'indoor' fire.

After eating invite people to sit around the fire and pass round a talking stick. Whoever holds the stick speaks of their personal harvest this year. When they have finished they say "I have spoken" and the talking stick is passed on to the next person. This allows each person a moment's review and the opportunity to share this with each other. Further conversations and networking can grow from this in the socialising that follows.

Making a Talking Stick, page 240

• Ask everyone to bring something that represents their own personal harvest. Sit in a circle around a beautiful cloth with a bowl of seasonal fruit at the centre.

Each person speaks about what they have brought and what they have learnt from it and then places it on the cloth. Give everyone full appreciation for their achievements but avoid getting into conversations. One person sounds a chime to bring the focus back if this does happen. Further conversations and networking can follow in the socialising time afterwards.

• Ask everyone to bring anything they have in abundance, either garden produce, seeds or things they have made, giving people the opportunity in the circle to share a bit about what they have bought and celebrate them together. Provide baskets for 'Baskets of Abundance' and when all is gathered in invite people to help themselves.

• Personal Review – Take a moment to think about your personal harvest and write about it in your journal. Make a list of all that has come to fruition this year, both physically and in your heart.

• What unexpected things happened that helped you?

• What happened that was difficult? What helpful gifts or seeds are hidden within this?

• From this review what new insights and understanding are emerging? First Impressions! Are any new directions presenting themselves? These are your new seeds to nurture during the winter. Like all seeds they need to incubate in the dark, in our fertile imaginations where they need time to take shape.

If you are with others, have a 'go round' and share your insights.

• Follow through with some further reflections.

What do your seeds need in order to grow within you?

What will stop them growing?

What can you do to help them grow?

• Place some native bulbs in a bowl at the centre of the circle. Each takes a bulb and names something they plan to nurture in the dark of the winter months. You might choose to have several rounds of this so everyone has a few bulbs to plant.

• In order to grow our new seeds, good compost is essential. We can begin making compost straight away by letting go of anything that is no longer serving us such as old outworn separation-thinking patterns and our fears for the future. Throw them all on the compost heap of regeneration. Learn to see chaos and disintegration as part of a healthy ecosystem. As the old breaks down, the compost this creates becomes the fertile edge from which something new can grow. Name what you let go of with great power and resolve!

• Trees are letting go of their leaves, reminding us to do the same, and to move into the winter free of the things that we no longer need, the things that block our happiness or inhibit our new ways forward.

Each person collects some autumn leaves and gathers round a central fire. Each names what they are letting go of and throws a leaf in the fire. You can have several rounds of this as often understanding deepens and more layers are revealed. It is also an opportunity for some light-hearted casting off, although there is always some truth revealed.

• What would you do for the healing of the Earth if you couldn't fail?

What particular projects could you start within the year?

What resources do you have, inner and outer, to help with this project?

What resources, inner and outer, will you need to encourage in yourself?

What could sabotage you, preventing you from achieving your goal?

How could you overcome these obstacles?

What can you do in the next 48 hours to achieve this goal? Make a commitment to do this.

Making a Talking Stick

Any native wood can be used for making a Talking Stick. You may decide to cut a special stick or a piece of wood may present itself either from your garden prunings or you may find a branch or tree blown down whilst out walking. To avoid working with old rotten wood, the rule is to only use wood that still has distinguishable leaves attached to it.

You could make several Talking Sticks, for different occasions and different uses. Each of the native trees has a different energetic signature and this becomes part of the energy of the Talking Stick.

SILVER BIRCH
New start. Boldness to begin. Overcoming difficulties. Cleansing.

ROWAN
Strong life force. Protection. Divination. Lightness of being.

WILLOW
Intuition. Dreaming. Releasing blocked feelings and emotions.

ALDER
Balance. Fire and Water. Male and Female. Connection to nature spirits.

ASH
Connecting the inner and outer. Unity. Past, present and future as one.

HAWTHORN
Listening to the heart. Giving and receiving love. Help from nature spirits.

OAK
Inner strength. Renewed potency. Courage.

HOLLY
Clear direction. Inner wisdom. Transforming negative emotions.

HAZEL
Divining truths from within. Transformation.

CRAB APPLE
Love. Inspiration. Abundance.

BLACKTHORN
Seeing things a different way. Choice.

N.B. A scratch from the thorns of blackthorn can cause septicemia.

YEW

The Ancestors. Death and rebirth. Regeneration.

N.B. The bark, leaves, wood and seed are poisonous.

ELDER

Letting go of the old. Endings and new beginnings. Throwing off congestion.

Before cutting wood be sure to check in with your heart and the tree first to see if it feels right. Thank the tree both before and after cutting. You may be lucky to find a natural 'twister', which has a natural spiral up the shaft created by honeysuckle.

After you have cut your stick, spend a little time with the tree as the shock settles. Meditate with your stick, intuiting its message to you and setting your intention to use it as a Talking Stick.

Follow steps 3-8 in the guide for making a staff or walking stick, see Finding and Crafting Your Own Staff or Walking Stick, page 215

You may decide to leave your Talking Stick plain or decorate with natural beads, threads, bone, bells or birds feathers, depending on what has significance and meaning for you. You may decide to carve it or paint it with symbols, or embed crystals or semi precious stones in the wood. This all helps to personalise and strengthen your relationship with your Talking Stick.

Making Home Made Incense from Native Plants

Coltsfoot, Birch Bark, Mugwort, Meadowsweet, Hops, Juniper leaves and berries, Rowan berries, Hawthorn berries, Heather, Rosehips, Rose petals, Pine needles, cones and sap, Yarrow

1. Gather herbs and berries on fine dry days and leave in labelled brown paper bags to dry out thoroughly, giving the bags a stir every day at the beginning to keep the air circulating. I often put aside herbs I am cutting back at this time of the year for this purpose. They don't need to be perfect as when making medicines.

2. When they are fully dry crumble them up finely, bag and label. Tree sap is collected in the spring and dried on an oiled piece of glass or slate.

3. The herbs are then burnt on charcoal wedges or your own charcoal. They can be burnt on a flat stone, in a stoneware dish or in a large shell. You can burn them singularly for specific uses or make combinations for different occasions.

BIRCH
Sap, leaves and bark. Use to honour and invoke new beginnings.

COLTSFOOT
This will help the mix to burn and the smoke is beneficial to the lungs.

CRAB APPLE
The wood, wood shavings and bark are all sweet smelling. Use for invoking self worth, and to value our own abundance; to help us count our blessings and to give generously of the love in our hearts.

MUGWORT
A powerful herb associated with inner strength, seeing clearly with the inner eye, dreams, visions and clairvoyance.

MEADOWSWEET
Associated with Lammas, meadowsweet is strengthening and soothing, brings relaxation, and openness, helping release fears and rigidity.

HOPS
Hop flowers help to ease the way through life's transitions and is soothing and calming.

JUNIPER

Use the wood, bark, leaves and the dried berries. Juniper brings personal power and helps us to get in touch with our vital forces, breaking through old patterns and bringing focus, new directions and increased connection to the web of life.

ROWAN BERRIES

Rowan strengthens positive life energy and personal power, bringing protection from negative influences. Brings a lightness of being and lifts the spirits.

HAWTHORN BERRIES

Hawthorn releases blocked energy and to open the heart to giving and receiving love. Increases our willingness to let go and trust.

ROSEHIPS, PETALS AND BUDS

Cut the rosehips help us to take out the fine hairs before drying. Rosehips help us to strengthen our ability to love ourselves as well as other people. Compassion. Forgiveness. Sensuality.

PINE

Use the bark, leaves, cones or sap. Pine brings the overview, clarity and insights.

HEATHER

Lifts the spirits and helps us find our true selves and our heart's desire. Helps to connect to the universal good and see beyond our own problems.

LAVENDER

Calming and restorative, strengthens the solar plexus and gives the power of discrimination and protection from unwanted influences.

ROSEMARY

Stimulating and energetic, moving energy along, bringing joy and strengthening purpose.

SAGE

A traditional burning herb that cleanses and heals blocked expression. Helps release and express feeling through the voice, as well as through crying and laughing.

THYME

An active herb for contacting the warrior within. It brings courage, bravery, and a sense of purpose.

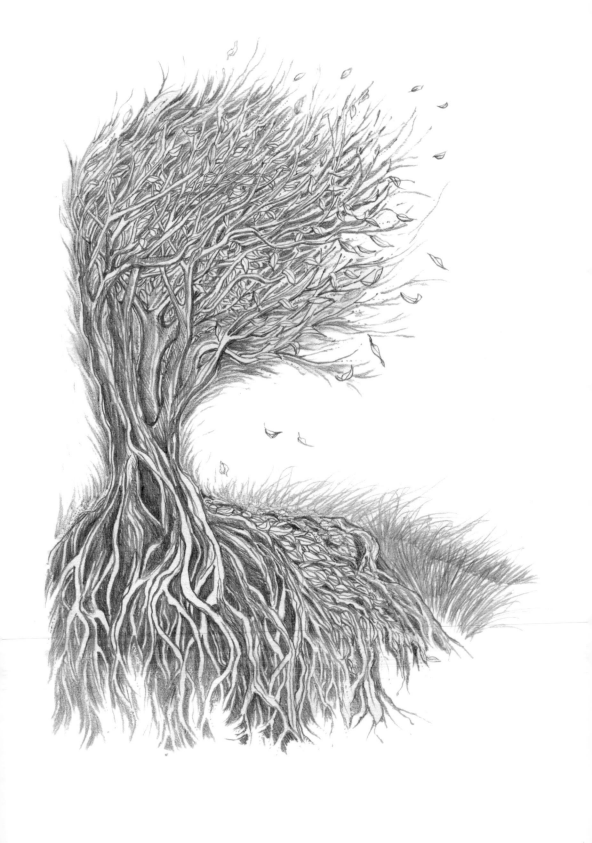

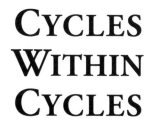

CYCLES
WITHIN
CYCLES

A book is a linear creature and the only way it becomes a circle is if you, dear reader, go back to the beginning. In this seasonal section this is easy, as the seasonal cycles continue on, never ending, year in year out, influencing our lives and bringing an ever-deepening connection and love for the Earth. So find your way back to the beginning of Part Two to the Edge of Winter on page and begin again with another new cycle. Each returning adds another layer of understanding to our journey of reconnection and renewal, taking us further into our appreciation and love for the infinite wonder and perfection of the Earth and the interconnected web of life that we are all blessed to be part of.

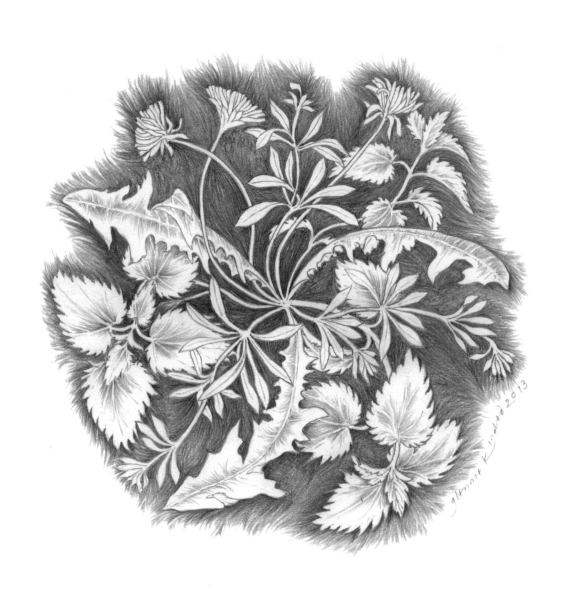

PLANT REFERENCE GUIDE OF NATIVE PLANTS AND TREES

These are some of the most useful wild native plants and trees that I have let into my garden and a reference guide to the plants covered in this book.

ANNUALS
Annuals have a life cycle of one year. They produce their own seeds and will self-seed or you can collect their seeds to re-grow the following spring.

PERENNIALS
Once perennials are established, the same plant will live for many years, and continues to make seed and self-seed each year.

BIENNIALS
Biennials take two years to complete the same cycle and don't flower the first year. They too will self-seed.

Betony (*Stachys officinalis*)

A native perennial, sometimes known as wood betony, it grows in woodland clearings, along hedgerows, grasslands and heaths. Flowers June to September.

In the Garden – An attractive garden plant with many medicinal uses. Sow the seeds in the spring.

Parts Used – Leaves and flowers.

Herbal Uses – Betony is a great cure-all, healing and strengthening the whole system, both physically and at a subtle level. It is a nerve tonic and a restoring herb and will help bring peaceful sleep if taken at bed time. Use for anxiety, nervous headaches, to bring clarity and relaxation. It has a beneficial effect on all digestive upsets, soothing and calming the whole of the digestive tract. It improves the memory and is perfect to take in our older years as a general restorer whenever we feel out-of-sorts. It improves the circulation. Use an infusion or oil made from the leaves for bathing bruises, sprains, haemorrhoids and varicose veins.

N.B. Do not take if pregnant.

Metaphysical Use – To help us become more instinctive and stay grounded. Moving us from our fears to a place of inner peacefulness.

In the Kitchen – Pick to dry for herb teas as it is coming into flower; make into tincture or add to elixirs; make a herbal oil; Add to herbal sleep pillows.

Drying Herbs, page 42
Making Tinctures, page 46
Elixirs, page 48
Herbal Oils, page 53
Herb Pillows, page 206

Chickweed (*Stellaria media*)

A native annual found growing everywhere. Also known as star weed because of its little white star flowers and winter weed because it grows throughout the winter.

In the Garden – If you have chickweed then encourage it, as it is a great winter salad plant. The more you pick, the more you get. Transplant new plants into containers near the house in the summer for a continuous autumn, winter and spring crop.

Parts Used – Leaves (and flowers).

Herbal Uses – This is a great spring tonic-herb, a supreme healer and restorer of the blood; use for cleansing the whole system. Eat regularly throughout the spring when it is at its best. Its action is cooling and soothing. Eat or drink regularly for digestive upsets and any hot inflammatory problems with the liver, kidneys and lungs. Use the infusion or oil for burns and to cleanse and to draw out poisons from any inflamed skin conditions.

Metaphysical Use – It enhances compassion and receptivity to others.

In the Kitchen – It is high in vitamins A and C and high in iron, copper, magnesium and calcium. Add to green smoothies, sandwiches, spinach-type mixes, soups, risottos, stir-fries, sprinkle over potatoes. Avoid using during summer as the stalks become stringy.

Making Tinctures, page 46
Chickweed Oil, page 148
Nettle and Chickweed Pesto, page 142
Green Smoothies, page 141

Chives (*Allium schoenoprasum*)

A native bulb, now rare in the wild, found on limestone. Flowers June to July.

In the Garden – An attractive plant that does well in containers. Grow from seed or by dividing existing clumps in the spring or autumn. This is an early salad plant that can be used from February onwards. Cut and use the flowers to improve the leaf quality.

Parts Used – Leaves and flowers.

Herbal Uses – A general tonic and cleanser, rich in iron, use for anaemia and as an antiseptic.

In the Kitchen – Greatly under estimated and under used in the kitchen. The leaves have a delicate onion flavour and the flowers are delicious. Chop up the leaves and use in salads and any egg, cheese or fish dish, in herb butters and dips. Break up the flowers and sprinkle as a last minute garnish.

Chive Oil, page 140
Edible Greens, page 140
Green Dip, page 143
Green Mayonnaise, page 144
Flower Vinegars, page 164
Flower Tinctures, page 185

Cleavers (*Galium aparine*)

A native annual found in hedges, woods, scrubland and waste ground. Commonly known as sticky willy or goosegrass. Flowers May to August.

In the Garden – The early tops are so delicious and it is such a good tonic and cleanser that it is worth having available in the garden. Collect the seeds and grow in a large container outside your door, where you can crop it frequently. Once it begins to grow long and flower, wrap it around itself so that the seeds fall in the container.

Parts Used – Leaves, especially the shooting tops.

Herbal Uses – A prime spring tonic and nutrient-packed herb. It strengthens and stimulates the lymphatic system, improves the immune system and fluid balance and dissolves undigested fats in the body. It is a blood purifier, cleanser and diuretic. Use when lymph nodes are enlarged, for skin eruptions, ulcers and tumours that are the result of poor lymph drainage. Take after viral infections, antibiotics, chemotherapy, steroids and anti depressants. Soothes all mucus membranes: the mouth, gut, vagina, and bladder (cystitis). Apply the juice from crushed plants directly on skin problems and insect bites, or make into an oil.

Metaphysical Use – It is soothing on emotions, bringing renewed strength and energy. Take before a change in direction.

In the Kitchen – Eat the leaf tops in salads every day whenever you can or add them to spinach mixes. They can also be juiced and added to green smoothies. Cut leaf tops in the spring and dry for teas, make into tincture and make an oil.

The Spring Tonic Herbs, page 138
Drying Herbs, page 42
Making Leaf Tincture, page 46
Infused Oils, page 53

Comfrey (*Symphytum officinale*)

A native perennial found in damp places, in ditches, along streams and river edges. Also known as knitbone and bruisewort. The flowers vary in colour from mauve, pinks and white. Flowers May to October.

N.B. Make sure that you have the true native as there are introduced comfreys that look similar and are high in pyrrolizidine alkaloid, which is toxic to the liver in large doses.

In the Garden – Worth growing in the garden as a plant fertiliser and to add to compost. Lay the leaves under seed potatoes as you plant them. Cultivate from seed or root division in the autumn. It does spread but is easy to pull up and compost.

Parts Used – Leaves. The root is now only used by a trained practitioner.

Herbal Uses – Use the fresh leaves as an infusion, mashed poultice (place on a piece of muslin), or infused oil. Use for varicose veins, surgical scars, bruises, sprains, torn ligaments and to mend broken bones (once they have been set by a professional). Drink the infusion as well as use it to bathe the skin but do not use directly on an open wound. Bathe around it. It will heal in record time so be sure the wound is clean.

N.B. Do not take internally if pregnant, breast feeding or have any problems with your liver.

Metaphysical Use – To help heal deep emotional traumas, particularly where there is a raw or sensitive wound in the psyche. For helping to cutting the ties that bind us to the past or another person.

In the Kitchen – Add to green spinach mixtures but eat in moderation. The flowering tops are rich in B12.

Comfrey Oil, page 140
Making Liquid Fertilisers, page 182

Corn Salad (*Valerianella locusta*)

A native annual found along hedge banks and roadsides. Also known as lambs lettuce. Flowers April to June.

In the Garden – A good garden plant as they are low growing and provide early spring salad leaves. They grow well in containers. They can be picked as early as February, especially if grown under cloches during the winter. Eventually they go to flower and then to seed. Collect the seeds and sow in the autumn for a winter and spring crop or sow in spring for a summer crop. Crop them by taking out the whole of the inner floret of leaves. Wash them well to get out the soil that always seems to lurk at the base of them. Leave the plant in the ground and another two smaller florets will grow in their place, giving you a second crop that can be picked a few weeks later.

Parts Used – Leaves.

Herbal Uses – Spring tonic.

In the Kitchen – Early spring edible leaves. It has a mild flavour, which mixes well with the stronger tastes of some of the other native plants that are around at this time.

Edible Natives, page 27
Edible Greens, page 140
Sowing Native Winter Greens, page 225

Cowslip (*Primula veris*)

A native perennial found on hedge banks, in meadows and along edges. Flowers April to May. A protected plant in the wild.

In the Garden – Grow from seed and split the clumps in the autumn. They will also self-seed. Give them to friends and plant them back in the wild.

Parts Used – Flowers.

Herbal Uses – A general tonic for the nervous system and of prime use for anxiety, stress, nervous headaches, and as a sedative. Drink before bed for insomnia. Use for neuralgia and as a detoxifying remedy, effective for colds, flu, fevers and coughs. Soothing to the skin and for sunburn.

Metaphysical Use – For when feeling vulnerable, for emotionally congested states, irritability and to lift the spirits.

In the Kitchen – Only pick your own cowslips from the garden.

Flower and Leaf Tinctures, page 46
Infused Herbal Oils, page 53
Flower Cordials, page 165
Flower Wines, page 166
Growing Cowslips, page 202

Crab Apple (*Malus sylvestris*)

A native tree of hedgerows and woods, identified by its thorns. Flowers in May and fruits in September.

In the Garden – A lovely wild garden tree, with blossom in the spring and fruit to use in the autumn. Plant the seeds or move trees in the autumn.

Parts Used – Petals and fruit

Herbal Uses – Apples are a tonic and cleanser, anti-inflammatory and antiseptic, the pectin in apple is a good germicide and promotes the growth of new skin tissue, providing a basis for the folk-cure of rubbing warts with two halves of an apple and then burying them. A poultice made from the boiled or roasted fruit will remove burn marks from the skin and is good for sore or inflamed eyes.

Metaphysical Use – For invoking self worth, and to value our own abundance, count our blessings and to give generously of the Love in our hearts. The flower essence can be used directly on the skin or in the bath to cleanse the skin and wounds. It can also be taken in water to lift a hangover.

In the Kitchen – Sprinkle the petals over salad. Crab apples can be used on their own and mixed with other fruit.

Crab Apple and Blackberry Wine, page 208
Crab Apple Jelly, page 235

Dandelion (*Taraxacum officinale*)

A common native perennial, found in grasslands and hedgerows. Flowers March to September.

In the Garden – Every gardener moans about dandelions but by using the leaves and flowers and saving the roots to dig up in the autumn for medicine or food, they take on a different significance in our gardens. Early leaves can be forced under plant pots, which are wrapped with straw or bubble wrap.

Parts Used – Leaves, flowers and roots.

Herbal Uses – Dandelion is a master healer, supporting overall health by flushing out toxins and improving the function of the liver, gall bladder, the kidneys, the urinary system and the digestive system. It is a prime lymph tonic, removing poisons from the system and cleansing the blood. It has a beneficial action on the lungs, helping coughs and bronchitis and will strengthen lung tissue. It helps reduce high blood pressure, high cholesterol, joint pains, viral infections, fluid retention, arthritis and hormonal imbalance. It is naturally high in potassium. The leaves are best for the kidneys and the roots for the liver.

Metaphysical Use – It brings determination and adaptability, clears emotional stagnation, turning depression into expression and self-empowerment.

In the Kitchen – A great spring tonic herb. Add the small young leaves to salad mixtures or to cooked leaf mixes. Take out the central stem of larger leaves to reduce their bitterness. The flower petals can be sprinkled on salads and any other food as a garnish, made into syrup, cordial and wine. Make the roots into tincture, a coffee type drink and beer, or dry for decoctions. Roots can also be chopped and fried and are sweetest in the autumn.

Spring Green Pickle, page 121
Edible Flowers, page 161
Infused Herbal Oils, page 53
Herbal and Flower Syrups, page 163
Flower Cordials, page 165

Flower Wine, page 166
Digging up and drying Roots, page 82
Making Root Tinctures, page 82
Dandelion and Burdock Beer, page 83
Dandelion Coffee, page 84

Elder *(Sambucus nigra)*

A common native shrub found in woods, waste grounds, hedgerows and disturbed ground. Flowers May to June. Fruits August to November. Steeped in folklore and myth requiring us to give thanks to the tree before cutting and gathering.

In the Garden – A good edge and hedge tree. Grow from cuttings or transplant young trees from seeds spread by birds.

Parts Used – Leaves, flowers, berries.

Herbal Uses – Once known as the country medicine chest because of its many uses. Drink an infusion of the flowers as a daily spring tonic and also as an expectorant to throw off excess mucus in head or lungs, for coughs, sinusitis, catarrh and hay fever. An infusion of the flowers makes a cooling lotion for the skin or for bathing tired eyes and drunk before bed are a sedative to help sleep. Fresh leaves can be rubbed on rashes, wounds, burns, sprains and bruises and as an insecticide, or made into a herbal oil. The berries are a wonderful restorative and will boost the immune system and ward off a cold, relieve coughs, sore throat, swollen glands and help a fever to break.

Metaphysical Use – For emotionally congested states, to move fears and bring clarity and wisdom.

In the Kitchen – Here are some of the things you can make with elder.

Edible Flowers, page 161
Infused Herbal Oils, page 53
Herbal and Flower Syrups, page 163
Elderflower Cordial, page 165
Flower Wines, page 166
Drying Flowers, page 162
Flower Tinctures, page 162
Herbal Honeys, page 51
Herb pillow, page 206

Drying Berries, page 231
Fruit Tinctures, page 231
Elderberry Elixir, page 232
Elderberry Syrup, page 233
Elderberry Wine, page 234
Elderberry Brandy, page 235
Elderberry and Apple Jam, page 236
Growing Trees from Cuttings, page 80
Making Elder Beads, page 91

Garlic Mustard (*Alliaria petiolata*)

A native biennial known as jack-by-the-hedge, poor man's mustard and hedge garlic. Flowers April to June.

In the Garden – This is a happy edge plant that likes the hedge bottoms. If you let it flower and seed will stick fairly well to its spot, but is easy to pull up or transplant depending on how much you like it.

Parts Used – Leaves.

Herbal Uses – Warms and strengthens digestion.

In the Kitchen – As garlic flavouring for salads, in sandwiches and sauces. Add to spinach type mixes, stews and soups.

Garlic Mustard Dip, page 143
Garlic Mustard Mayonnaise, page 143

Hawthorn (*Crataegus monogyna*)

A native shrub found in woods and hedgerows. Known as the may tree or white thorn. Flowers May to June. Fruits August to November.

In the Garden – A hedge plant that can be left to grow into a mature tree. Much loved by the birds. Grow from seed or dig up self seeded saplings.

Parts Used – Leaves, flowers and fruit (haws).

Herbal Uses – A safe and primary remedy for the heart, relieving palpitations, angina, hardening of the arteries, water retention and poor circulation. It has the ability to regulate high or low blood pressure depending on the need and will gently bring the heart to normal function. Use for any nervous conditions including stress and insomnia. A poultice of the pulped berries or leaves has strong drawing powers, and has long been used for embedded thorns, splinters and whitlows.

Metaphysical Use – Hawthorn has the ability on the subtle level to release blocked energy and to open the heart to giving and receiving love. By releasing stress it enhances the person's ability to let go and trust.

In the Kitchen – Eat the young leaves and flowers in salads. There are many ways to preserve and use the berries and the flowers.

Drying Flowers, page 162
Hawthorn Flower Tincture, page 162
Flower Syrups, page 163
Flower Cordials, page 165
Flower Wine, page 166
Drying Berries, page 231
Hawthorn Fruit Tincture, page 231
Fruit Syrups, page 232
Fruit Wine, page 207
Hawthorn Brandy, page 235

Hops (*Humulus lupulus*)

A native perennial, found in hedges and woodland edges. Flowers July to August.

In the Garden – Grow from seed or transplants.

Parts Used – Sprouting shoots, flowers.

Herbal Uses – For nervous tension and insomnia, drink an infusion of hop flowers at bed time or dry them and make a hop pillow. Drink as an infusion for lack of appetite, sluggish digestion, and as a liver tonic. Use the infusion externally for bruises, boils, neuralgia and rheumatic pains. They have an oestrogenic action, making them useful during the menopause. They will depress a man's libido, but have the opposite effect on women!

N.B. Do not take if you suffer from depression.

Metaphysical Use – Soothing and calming, Hops helps to ease the way through life's transitions.

In the Kitchen – Pick the shoots as soon as they appear and use in salads or they can be steamed and used like asparagus. Good in egg dishes. Dry for infusions, make into tincture, in calming elixirs and beer.

Drying Flowers, page 162
Herb Pillows, page 206
Making Tinctures, page 46
Hop Beer, page 209

Lady's Mantle (*Alchemilla filicaulis*)

A native perennial found on grasslands and wood edges, flowering May to September. The alchemists of old revered this plant, and collected the drop of water that magically appears each morning in the cup like leaves. This is not dew, but exudes from the plant itself and holds all the properties of the plant.

In the Garden – Grow from seed or self-seeded transplants. The roots can be divided in spring or autumn. It grows in poor soil, sun or part shade.

Parts Used – Leaves.

Herbal Uses – Known as a woman's herb, use as a general tonic to the reproductive organs and as a douche for any vaginal irritations. It will reduce period pains, regulate periods and is good for the menopause.

N.B. It is a uterine stimulant, so avoid if pregnant.

Metaphysical Use – To get in touch with our feminine sides, our intuition and the inspirations that feed our magical nature. It is both calming and restorative.

In the Kitchen – The young leaves are added to salads. Dry the leaves for infusions or make into a tincture or flower essence.

Making Tinctures, page 46
Honey Elixirs, page 48

Lady's Smock (*Cardamine pratensis*)

A native perennial found in damp meadows and stream edges. Flowers April to June. Known as cuckoo flower or bittercress.

In the Garden – A low-growing plant with beautiful delicate lilac flowers. Eat the leaves, flowers and flower buds in early spring. Prevent from flowering to increase the leaf yield. Grow from seed in spring, or transplant and split the plants.

Parts Used – Leaves and flowers.

Herbal Uses – A spring tonic high in vitamin C, minerals and iron that aids digestion and restores lost appetite. It also can be used as an expectorant and is good for coughs. It will stimulate the circulation and is beneficial to the heart.

Metaphysical Use – Once known as the fairies' flower, it helps us become more finely tuned to the ethereal spirit of nature.

In the Kitchen – Add the leaves and flowers to salads, soups and green mixtures. It tastes rather like watercress.

Making Honey Elixirs, page 48
Iron Tonic Elixir, page 50
Flower vinegars, page 164

Mallow, common (*Malva sylvestris*)

A native perennial found in all *edge* places. Flowers June to September.

In the Garden – Grow from seed. It will self-seed along hedge bottoms.

Parts Used – Leaves, flowers and fruit.

Herbal Uses – Mallow is soothing and healing to the respiratory and urinary systems and will reduce inflammation. Make a tincture or an infusion of leaves and flowers for sore throats, coughs, colds, stomach ulcers, stomach upsets and indigestion. Make a poultice or an infused oil for boils, bruises, sprains, muscular aches and pains, scalds, burns, sunburn, insect bites and stings (or use the bruised fresh leaves or infusion). For toothache and sore gums, chew a few young leaves and flowers that have previously been softened for a few minutes in some boiling water and drink the water.

Metaphysical Use – For smooth communication, helping us to be open and warm towards all life and all people.

In the Kitchen – Add the petals, young leaves and flat seeds (called 'cheeses') to salads or pick as a tasty nibble while out walking.

Mallow Tincture, page 185
Mallow Oil, page 186

Mints

There are over two hundred different varieties of mint in this country. These three are considered to be our true natives:

Apple-Scented Mint (*Mentha rotundifolia*)
A native perennial found along roadsides and in ditches. Flowers July to October.

Corn Mint (*Mentha arvensis*)
A native perennial found in woods, fields and damp places also known as lambs mint because it is eaten with lamb. Flowers May to October.

Water Mint (*Mentha aquatica*)
A native perennial found in damp places, along riverbanks, streams, marshes and fens. Flowers July to October.

In the Garden – A new plant will grow from even a tiny bit of the root. Grow it in a container or confine it with well dug in tiles or bricks, unless you are happy for it to take over an area. Grows vigorously from early spring. Cut and dry the first crop just before the flowers open, so you have mint for the winter. Plenty more will grow for fresh mint teas until autumn.

Parts Used – Leaves.

Herbal Uses – Drink the tea as a digestive tonic, for nausea, acidity and for any problems in the mouth.

In the Kitchen – Add the early mint tops to salads. Use as a garnish and cake decoration. Cut and dry for herb teas, make into a tincture or as an ingredient in digestive elixirs.

Drying Herbs, page 42
Mint Leaf Tincture, page 138
Digestive Tonic Elixir, page 50
Mint Honey, page 188
Making Elixirs, page 48

Mullein (*Verbascum thapsus*)

A native biennial, found growing on sunny banks, disturbed ground and waysides, also known as Aaron's rod, hags taper and torch plant. It has beautiful fragrant flowers, which begin at midsummer and gradually work their way up the flowering stalk. In the past the finished spikes were dried, dipped in fat or oil and used as a slow-burning taper or torch.

In the Garden – Mullein is a tall, striking plant that likes dry ground. Grow from seed and allow it to self-seed along the wild edges.

Parts Used – Leaves, flowers.

Herbal Uses – The leaves and flowers are good for the lungs, the throat and the lymphatic system. Make into tea or tincture for all mucus congestion, respiratory infections, bronchial infections, coughs, asthma, and glandular imbalance. It calms and strengthens the digestive system and the nerves. Make a herbal oil from the flowers and use for ear ache to reduce the pain and fight infection. Use the fresh leaves or infusion to draw out splinters. Previously the leaves were dried and used in country tobacco.

Metaphysical Use – Use to clear stuck energy, find clarity and affirm your higher purpose.

In the Kitchen – Make oil from the flower buds and flowers. Dry the leaves or make into tincture or elixir.

Drying Flowers, page 162
Making Flower Tinctures, page 185
Mullein Oil, page 186
Cough Elixir, page 50

Nettle (*Urtica dioica*)

A native perennial that grows on disturbed ground, in woods, ditches and grassy places. Flowers May to September.

In the Garden – A wonderful attractor of insects. It has a creeping root, which can be contained. Keep a patch as a crop and cut to the base frequently to ensure fresh tops and to stop it going to flower and seed. Make into a crop fertiliser.

Parts Used – The fresh young tops.

Herbal Uses – Collect nettle tops in the spring when they are at their best. A prime blood tonic and blood purifier, rich in iron and minerals.

Metaphysical Use – Nettle brings a fiery determination and encourages us to keep our boundaries.

In the Kitchen – A good vegetable with a high mineral content that can be added to all spinach mixtures – but only use the young tops. Dry nettle tops for a tonic tea or make into a tincture as an iron tonic or add to iron tonic elixirs.

Drying Herbs, page 42
Nettle Tincture, page 138
Iron Tonic Elixir, page 50
Nettle Soup, page 142
Nettle and Chickweed Pesto, page 142
Making Herbal and Flower Syrups, page 163

Red Clover (*Trifolium pratense*)

A native perennial found in fields and growing in grass. Flowers May to September.

In the Garden – A nitrogen-fixer that will enrich the soil. Sow from seed.

Parts Used – Leaves and flowers.

Herbal Uses – A prized herbal remedy, known to be restorative and valued for its alkaline property and its beneficial influence on cancers. It assists the lymph system, cleanses the blood, promotes expectoration of mucus from the body, soothes the nerves and helps promote sleep. Mix the flowers with honey for coughs.

In the Kitchen – The early leaves can be used in salads or added to cooked meals. Break the flowers up and sprinkle in salads. Make into tincture and dry for herb teas. Only pick the youngest most perfect flowers, and avoid any that have browned at the edges.

Drying Flowers, page 162
Red Clover Syrup, page 163
Making Flower Vinegars, page 164
Flower Cordials, page 165
Red Clover Tincture, page 185
Red Clover Honey, page 188
Candied Flowers, page 188

Rose, wild (*Rosa canina*)

A native shrub that flowers June to July with rosehips in September.

In the Garden – Let this delightful plant ramble on your wild edges. Trim back every autumn to keep it in check.

Parts Used – Petals and fruit (rosehips).

Herbal Uses – The petals and the rosehips are an immune system support, rich in vitamin C. They are diuretic and help clear out toxins. They are cooling to all hot conditions. Use for colds and flu, sore throats and viral infections. Use as a heart tonic, a hormonal balancer and a tonic for the female reproductive system.

N.B. Do not internalise the hairy seeds of the hips.

Metaphysical Use – To help you to love yourself and strengthen your loving heart.

In the Kitchen – Shake off the petals so that the rosehips can form and add them to salads and to sandwiches. Use for wine, syrups, honeys and cordials. Other scented rose petals can also be added to your creations. Pick the vitamin and mineral-rich rosehips in the autumn. Cut them open while soft and scoop out the hairy seeds and dry for teas or for making tincture.

Flower Wine, page 166
Flower Syrups, page 163
Rose Petal Tincture, page 185
Infused Flower Oils, page 186
Rose Petal Honey, page 188
Candied Flowers, page 188
Rosehip Tincture, page 231
Rosehip Syrup, page 232
Fruit Honeys, page 233
Fruit Wine, page 207
Fruit Brandy, page 235

Rowan (*Sorbus aucuparia*)

A native tree found in woods and mountains, also known as mountain ash. Flowers May to June. Fruits August to September.

In the Garden – An attractive small garden tree that can be coppiced.

Parts Used – Fruit – which must be cooked.

Herbal Uses – The jam or jelly is astringent (contracts tissue) and good for mild diarrhoea. It strengthens the immune system and cleanses the blood.

Metaphysical Use – Strengthens positive life energy and personal power, bringing protection from negative influences. Brings a lightness of being and lifts the spirits.

In the Kitchen – Mix with other fruit and use for making jams, jellies and wine.

Drying Berries and Fruit, page 231
Fruit Syrups, page 232
Fruit Honeys, page 233
Rowan Wine, page 207
Rowan Brandy, page 235
Rowan Berry Jelly, page 235

Salad Burnet (*Sanguisorba minor*)

A native perennial found in meadows and dry pastures. Flowers May to August.

The flowers, called red knobs in Nottinghamshire, are very unusual as the flowers at the top of the flower ball are female, those in the middle are hermaphrodite and those at the bottom are male. They have no nectar to attract insects but rely on the pollen being carried by the wind.

In the Garden – This is an attractive garden salad plant that grows throughout the winter. It grows well in containers and at the front of borders. Sow seeds in seed trays in the spring or autumn and plant out when they are big enough to handle. They fan from the middle and a mature plant needs a good 30cm diameter, less if it is kept cropped. Its unusual flowers need picking if you are using it as a salad plant. Let one or two plants flower just to enjoy them and to save seed for re-sowing.

Parts Used – Leaves.

In the Kitchen – An all year salad plant that tastes a bit like cucumber. The leaves become bitter as soon as the flowers form so keep picking the flowers whenever they appear. Strip the leaves from the stalks. The more you pick the more fresh new leaves grow.

Edible Greens, page 140
Green Dips, page 143
Green Mayonnaise, page 144
Green Pesto, page 142
Sowing Native Winter Greens, page 225

Self Heal (*Prunella vulgaris*)

A native perennial found growing on the edge of woodlands and fields. Flowers June to September.

In the Garden – An attractive garden plant with bright purple flowers, much loved by the bees. It grows well from seed and it transplants well. It will grow well in containers and once established it will self-seed.

Parts Used – The flower heads.

Herbal Uses – A restorative that stimulates the immune system. It clears liver stagnation and is antiviral. Good for fevers, flu, colds and throat problems. A prime wound herb for sores, ulcers, and piles. A good mouthwash or throat gargle.

Metaphysical Use – To open ourselves to our own healing and our spiritual path. It brings the gift to speak our own truth and communicate from the heart.

In the Kitchen – Pick and dry the flower heads as they come into flower (leave some for their seeds), or make them into tinctures, elixirs and infused oil.

Immune System Booster Elixir, page 50
Restored Energy Elixir, page 50
Drying Flowers, page 162
Flower Tinctures, page 185
Infused Flower Oils, page 186

Sorrel (Rumex acetosa)

A native perennial found in grassland, in pastures and along roadsides. It has distinctive small arrow shaped leaves, which have a sharp lemony flavour. They can be picked as early as February. It flowers May to June.

In the Garden – Grow as a vegetable crop. It likes a damp position. Sow the seeds in September or March and thin out as the plants form. Ready to pick in July. Once established in your garden the leaves can be picked from February to May. Prevent from flowering to increase the leaf yields. Cut back frequently to encourage new young shoots for salads. The roots can be divided in the autumn and placed in new positions about a foot apart.

Parts Used – Leaves.

Herbal Uses – The leaves contain binoxalate of potash, also present in rhubarb, which gives its sharp acidy flavour, and should be avoided by those with rheumatic conditions.

In the Kitchen – Add the leaves to salad, or make a green sauce with a sharp lemony flavour, which is traditionally eaten with fish. Add to any spinach-type mixtures.

Green Dip, page 143
Green Mayonnaise, page 144
Green Pesto, page 142
Sowing Native Winter Greens, page 225

St Johns Wort (*Hypericum perforatum*)

A native perennial found in grassland and hedgerows. Flowers June to September.

In the Garden – Grow from seed or transplant self-seeded plants.

Parts Used – Flowers.

Herbal Uses – A prime nerve tonic used to treat damage to nerve endings such as burns and wounds. It is also a mood enhancer that will relieve stress, anxiety and lift the spirits. Use for M.E./chronic fatigue syndrome, S.A.D., mild depression and jet lag. It is a diuretic that rids the body of toxins and tones the urinary system. It strengthens the digestive system and the liver and is an antibacterial, antiviral and an analgesic that helps reduce pain. Use the oil externally for sciatica, shingles, backache, headache, rheumatic pain, to heal and soothe burns, cuts, sores, varicose veins and ulcers and take the tincture at the same time.

N.B. If St Johns Wort is over-used it can increase sensitivity to the sun. Do not over-use if you are on allopathic medication, including the contraceptive pill. Do not use if you are pregnant. Do not use if you are taking anti-depressant drugs.

Metaphysical Use – A support through life's transitions, it lifts the spirits, reduces fear and oversensitivity. Traditionally used as a protection against harmful influences and to stand strong in the light.

In the Kitchen – Make a tincture and oil from the flowers. Traditionally these are picked at midday.

Drying Flowers, page 162
Flower Tinctures, page 185
Infused Flower Oils, page 186

Valerian (*Valeriana officinalis*)

A native perennial found growing on high pastures, dry heath lands and along roadsides. This plant has a very distinctive smell and tall white to pink flowers. Flowers June to August.

In the Garden – An attractive garden plant that grows to more than a metre high so plant at the back of borders and along hedges. Prevent the plants from flowering so the energy goes into the roots, which can be dug up every 2 or 3 years. Remove the largest white roots for making tincture and then replant.

Parts Used – The roots are best made into a tincture or soaked as a cold decoction because of their pungent smell.

Herbal Uses – A nerve tonic for mental and nervous exhaustion and anxiety. It is a mild sedative that acts as a natural tranquiliser, improving sleep without affecting the ability to remember dreams or making you feel sluggish the next day. For nervous headaches, bile dysfunctions, stomach and intestinal cramps and painful periods. It has a calming effect on the heart. A painkiller for any condition that needs the whole system to relax.

N.B. A powerful herb that should not be used continually.

Metaphysical Use – It will help 'earth' you when you have become overwhelmed by fears or after a physical or mental trauma.

In the Kitchen – Make a tincture from the roots or dry the roots for cold decoctions.

Drying Roots, page 82
Root Tincture, page 82

Vervain (*Verbena officinalis*)

A native perennial that used to be common along roadsides and on dry grasslands. It was a sacred plant of the Druids, who would not pick it without due ceremony and giving thanks. Flowers June to September. Becoming rare in the wild.

In the Garden – An attractive garden plant with pale pink flowers that grows well in containers and self seeds. Grow from seed and then divide plants in the spring or autumn. Collect the seeds in autumn to re-sow the following spring. Such a valuable herb, so give them to friends and replant them out in the wild.

Parts Used – Leaves and flowers.

Herbal Uses – Known as a 'heal-all', it is a nerve tonic and mood enhancer and will lift the spirits. Use for nervous headaches, nervous exhaustion, stress, anxiety, M.E./chronic fatigue syndrome. Use for premenstrual tension and during the menopause. A liver, kidney and digestive tonic, which will eliminate toxins and balance thyroid function. It is soothing, cooling and healing. Apply the crushed leaf or an infusion to cuts and sores, burns and skin irritations. Will encourage sweating in fevers to keep down the temperature. Good for convalescence, especially in children, facilitating a time of calm, relaxed recuperation.

N.B. Avoid if pregnant or breast feeding.

Metaphysical Use – To help bring a calmer lifestyle to those who work too hard, are over stimulated, intense, strong-willed and can't relax.

In the Kitchen – Dry for teas and make into tincture and 'anti-stress' and 'feel-good' elixirs.

Drying Herbs, page 42
Honey Elixirs, page 48
Flower Tinctures, page 185
Herbal Honeys, page 51

Violet

Sweet Violet (*Viola odorata*)
A native perennial found in hedgerows, woods and damp places. This is the scented violet. Flowers February to April.

Dog violet (*Viola riviniana*)
A common native perennial found in hedgerows and wood edges. Flowers April to July.

In the Garden – A small but beautiful garden plant that grows well in containers and self-seeds in any nook and cranny. Sow the seeds in the autumn.

Parts Used – Leaves and flowers.

Herbal Uses – It is cooling and soothing wherever there is heat and inflammation. A cleanser that helps to clear toxins, moves mucus, good for coughs and upper respiratory catarrh. Use for headaches, hangovers, depression and insomnia. Contains salicylates, which reduce inflammation in arthritis and rheumatism.

N.B. Do not use if sensitive to aspirin.

Metaphysical Use – It is soothing and healing and brings protection. Use to enhance openness, warmth and love.

In the Kitchen – All violets are edible. Use the flowers to decorate salads and other food. Use the sweet violet to flavour elixirs, cakes and drinks and for candied decorations.

Making Tinctures, page 46
Candied flowers, page 188
Growing Violets, page 202

Wintercress (*Barbarea vulgaris*)

A native biennial or perennial, also known as yellow rocket and land cress. An edge plant found along rivers, canals, roadsides and waste places. Flowers May to September.

In the Garden – The young seedlings grow throughout the winter and are a very early salad plant. Grows well in containers. Prevent most of the plants from flowering to use the leaves. Let the rest self-seed for the following year or save the seeds and sow in July.

Parts Used – Leaves.

Herbal Uses – Spring tonic.

In the Kitchen – A useful early salad plant that taste like watercress. Add to spinach-type mixes.

Edible Greens, page 140
Green Dips, page 143
Green Mayonnaise, page 144
Sowing Native Winter Greens, page 225

Yarrow (*Achillea millefolium*)

A common native perennial found in meadows and along roadsides. Also known as milfoil (a thousand leaves), and nosebleed on account of its ability to stop bleeding. Flowers June to November.

In the Garden – An attractive garden plant that flowers for a long time. Grow from seed and split established clumps.

Parts Used – Leaves.

Herbal Uses – Use the infusion for bathing wounds, inflammations and piles. The fresh leaf will stop bleeding. Yarrow combines well with elderflowers and mint to bring out a fever. Drink an infusion frequently for colds and flu.

In the Kitchen – Use the very young leaves in salad and add them to any green mixes for cooking. Dry the leaves for infusions. Make into tincture and make a herbal wound oil.

Drying Herbs, page 42
Flower and Leaf Tinctures, page 162
Infused Herbal Oils, page 53

RESOURCES AND RECOMMENDATIONS

BOOKS

Field Guides

Wild Flowers of Britain; Roger Phillips; Pan Books, 1994.
Wild Flowers of Britain and Northern Europe; Marjorie Blamey, Richard Fitter and Alistair Fitter; Collins, 1974.

Foraging and Wild Food

The Elder in History, Myth and Cookery; Ria Loohuizen; Cromwell Press, 2002.
Field Guide to Edible Mushrooms of Britain and Europe; Peter Jordan; New Holland Publishers, 2010.
Food for Free; Richard Mabey; Collins, 1972.
Hedgerow Cookbook; Glennie Kindred; Wooden Books, 1999.
The Hedgerow Handbook – Recipes, Remedies and Rituals; Adele Nozedar; Square Peg, 2012. Includes fabulous drawings by Lizzie Harper.
Wild Food; Roger Phillips; Pan Books, 1983.

Herb Books

The Complete Floral Healer; Annie McIntyre; Gaia Books, 1996.
The Healing Power of Celtic Plants – Their History, Their Use and the Scientific Evidence That They Work; Angela Paine; O Books, 2006.
Hedgerow Medicine; Julie Bruton-Seal and Mathew Seal; Merlin Unwin, 2008. My favourite herbal, full of sound herbal information, interesting facts and snippets, and more importantly it teaches you to think and act like a herbalist. www.hedgerowmedicine.com

Herbal Healers – 21 Familiar Kitchen and Garden Herbs; Glennie Kindred; Wooden Books, 1999.

Herbal Recipes for Radiant Health; Rosemary Gladstar; Storey Publishing, 2001.

The Holistic Herbal; David Hoffman; Findhorn Press, 1983.

The Illustrated Herbal Handbook; Juliette de Bairacli Levy; Faber and Faber, 1974. The great grandmother of modern herbalists, who sadly died a few years ago. She learnt from gypsy lore and her understanding of healing animals remains invaluable.

A Modern Herbal; Mrs M Grieve; Tiger Books International, 1981. First published 1933. The most comprehensive study still today and a must for all those interested in herbs and our native plants.

Practical Herbs; Henriette Kress; Yrtit ja yrttierapia Henriette Kress, 2011.

A Woman's Book of Herbs; Elizabeth Brooke; The Women's Press, 1992.

Other Inspirational Reading

Active Hope – How to Face the Mess We're In Without Going Crazy; Joanna Macy and Chris Johnstone; New World Library, 2012. www.activehope.info

Arborsculpture – Solutions For a Small Planet; Richard Reames; Aborsmith Studios, 2005. Growing chairs, dens and other fantastic things from living wood. www.arborsmith.com

The Art of the Mindful Gardener; Ark Redwood; Leaping Hare Press, 2011.

At Day's Close – Night in Times Past; A. Roger Ekirch; W.W. Norton and Company, 2005.

Earthing; Clinton Ober, Stephen T. Sinatra and Martin Zucker; Basic Health Publications Inc, 2010.

Sanctuary – Finding a New Relationship with the Land; Elizabeth Edwards, Fionnuala O'Hare, Kath Simmonds, Jill Taylor and Sue Weaver; Permanent Publications, 2002.

ORGANISATIONS

Association of Master Herbalists
www.associationofmasterherbalists.co.uk
The Herb Society
www.herbsociety.org.uk
The National Institute for Medical Herbalists (NIMH)
www.nimh.org.uk
Unified Register of Herbal Practitioners (URHP)
www.urp.com

Agroforestry Research Trust
www.agroforestry.co.uk
Plants for a Future
www.pfaf.org
Wild Plant Conservation
www.plantlife.org.uk
Taking Initiative For the Survival of the Honey Bee
www.beeguardian.org

NATIVE PLANT, SEED AND BULB SUPPLIERS

www.chilternseeds.co.uk
www.shiptonbulbs.co.uk
www.meadowmania.co.uk
www.wildflowersuk.com
www.englishplants.co.uk
www. suffolkherbs.com

HERB SUPPLIERS

The Organic Herb Trading Company
www.organicherbtrading.com

Star Child. Glastonbury
www.starchild.co.uk

FLOWER ESSENCE SUPPLIERS

The British Association of Flower Essence Producers
www.bafep.com

The Bach Flower Centre
www.bachcentre.com

Essences made with wild plants in wild places
www.wildmedicine.co.uk
Consultations and advice and the author's personal recommendation

SUNRISE AND SUNSET TIMES

The Earth Pathways Diary
All the sunrise and sunset, moonrise and moonset times every day for the UK,
along with a focus for each of the Earth Festivals, writing, painting and photos
to inspire our connection to the Earth.
www.earthpathwaysdiary.co.uk

Sunrise and sunset times world wide
www.timeanddate.com

BUYING DARK MEDICINE BOTTLES

www.naturallythinking.com
www.baldwins.co.uk

INSPIRING WEBSITES

www.dreamthefuture.org.uk
Sharing visions of positive futures to inspire and encourage each other to dare
to dream! Contact Marion McCartney through this website for more details
about Wonder Wanders.

www.eartheducation.org.uk
The Institute For Earth Education.

www.permaculture.co.uk
Permaculture magazine. Practical news and articles on permaculture, self sufficiency,
farming, gardening, small holding and sustainable living.

www.glenniekindred.co.uk
Includes a monthly focus on native plants and trees with recipes, more
information about my other books, magazine articles and details and dates
of future courses, workshops and talks.

http://theherbarium.wordpress.com
Blog for traditional herbalists in times of transition.

INDEX

absorbing herbs through the skin **52**
Achillea millefolium **280**
acidity, herbs 266, 269
acute conditions 45
Alchemilla filicaulis **263**
Alder 80, 204, 241
Alliaria petiolata **260**
Allium schoenoprasum **252**
ancestors, the 75
annuals 249
antibacterial herbs 275
antiseptic herbs 252
April into May **151-173**
archways, natural 64, 94
art of seeing, the 152
Ash 204, 241
Autumn 219-244
Autumn Equinox 54, 58, 220,
    237-244
Autumn, On the Edge of **195-217**

balance 10, 145, 146, 178, 224
Barbarea vulgaris **279**
barefoot walking **14**, 130
bathbag, making 206
bead necklace, making 147
Beech 167, 168
beech leaf gin 167
bees 29
beginnings, middles and endings 60
beginning a celebration 61
Beltain 54, 58, **169-173**
Betony 50, 206, 228, **250**
biennials 249
Birch, Silver 167, 168, 204, 241, 243
birds 29, 96
blackberries 200, 207, 232, 233
blackberry and crab apple wine 208
Blackthorn 84, 204, 241
blood cleansing herbs 229, 251, 253,
    258, 268, 269, 271
Borage 49, 188
Broom 165, 166
brain tonic elixir 50
bruises, herbs 250, 254, 259, 262
burns/sunburn, herbs 251, 256, 257,
    259, 265, 275, 277

candied flowers 188
Cardamine pratensis **264**
celebrations 55-67
celebrating outside 63
celebrating alone 65
Chamomile 49, 102, 206
Chickweed 50, 101, 115, 121, 131, 132,
    138, 139, 140, 141, 142, 148, 155,
    158, 202, **251**
chickweed oil 148
Chives 50, 119, 138, 139, 140, 141,
    161, 227, **252**
chive oil 140
chive flower vinegar 164
chronic conditions 45
circulation herbs 250, 261, 264
Cleavers 50, 102, 121, 131, 132, 139,
    140, 141, 142, 155, 201, 225, **253**
closing circles 62
co-creating celebrations 66
colds 50, 119,
colds/flu/viral infections, herbs 256, 259,
    265, 270, 273, 280
cold infusion 44
Coltsfoot 101, 114, 120, 130, 217, 243
Comfrey 130, 139, 140, 155, 254
comfrey oil 140
compost, making 203
commemorative tree planting 76
container gardening 118
cordials, making 165
Corn Salad 115, 132, 141, 201, 202,
    225, **255**
cough elixir 50
coughs 50, 101, 114, 119,
coughs, herbs 256, 258, 259, 264, 265,
    267, 269, 278
cough medicine, making 101, 119
Cowslip 49, 102, 161, 162, 165, 201, **256**
cowslip flower oil 163
cowslip, growing 202
Crab Apple 155, 200, 204, 207, 241,
    243, **257**
crab apple and blackberry wine 208
crab apple jelly, making 235
Cross Quarter Festivals 58
Crataegus monogyna **261**

Dandelion 50, 82, 84, 101, 115, 130, 132, 138, 140, 148, 155, 161, 163, 165, **258**
dandelion and burdock beer , making 83
dandelion coffee, making 84
dandelion flowers 163, 166
dandelion oil 148, 163
darkness, natural 220
dark medicine bottles, buying 284
dark storage jars, making 210
December into January 93-109
decoction **44**
depression, herbs 275, 277, 278
detox/diuretic herbs 253, 258, 270, 275, 277, 278
digestive elixir 50
digestive herbs 250, 251, 253, 262, 264, 265, 266, 267, 275, 276, 277
doorways, natural 64
door wreath, making 108
dosage guidelines 45
drawing and painting 152, 178, 202
drying berries and fruit 231
drying flowers 162, 185
drying herbs **42**, 43, 162, 185
drying roots 82

earache, herbs 267
Earth festivals, the 55-67, 86-91
Earth cycles, the 55-59
Earth spirit or Imbolc doll, making 125
edible leaves/edible greens 27, 40, 114, 115, 130, 132, **140**, 157, 161, 168
edible flowers 161
Elder 80, 91, 148, 204, 242, **259**
elder beads, making 91
elderflowers 49, 101, 102, 154, 161, 163, 165, 168, 188, 206
elderflower cordial 165
elderberries 50, 100, 119, 207, 231, 232, 233
elderberry and apple jam, making 236
elderberry brandy 235
elderberry and apple chutney, making 236
elderberry elixir , making 232
elderberry syrup, making 233
elderberry wine, making 234
Elder leaf oil 148, 163
electrical Earth **14**
elixirs, dosage 45
elixirs, making **48- 50**, 120, 139, 231
endings of celebrations 62
Equinoxes, the 57
Equinox, Spring, *see Spring Equinox*

Equinox, Autumn, *see Autumn Equinox*
evergreens, traditional native 105, 107,108
expectorant herbs 229, 259, 269, 269, 278
Eyebright 229
eyes, herbs 229, 257, 259

female reproductive system, herbs 263, 270, 276, 277
Fennel 139
fevers, herbs 256, 258, 277, 280
foraging **17**, 41, 77, 114, 130, 155, 180, 200, 223
foraging stick, making 222
flash mob 160
flower and leaf tinctures 162, 185,
flower essences, making **38**, 139, 154, 179
flower essence suppliers 283
flowers, candied 188
flower cordials 165
flowers, drying 162, 185
flowers, edible 161, 182
flower honeys 188
flower oils 186
flower syrups 163
flower vinegars 164
flower wines 166
foot baths 52, 101
fruit brandy 235
fruit chutneys, making 236
fruit, drying 231
fruit honeys 233
fruit jam and jelly, making 235
fruit, syrups 232
fruit, tinctures and elixirs 231
fruit vinegars 209
fruit wine **207**, 234

Galium aparine **253**
gardening, container 118
gardening, no-dig, 78
gardening, long term planning, 79
Garlic Mustard 130, 132, 140, 143, 155, **260**
garlic mustard mayonnaise 143
Garlic, Wild 131
greens, edible 140
green dips 143
green feta pie 141
green mayonnaise 144
green man / green woman mask, making 172

green pesto 142
green pie 141
green smoothie 141
green spinach-type mixtures 140
guerrilla gardening 31, 81, 98, 118, 136, 159, 183, 204, 230

Hairy Bittercress 132,140
hand soaks 52
hangovers, herbs 257, 278
Hawthorn 49, 50, 102, 130, 132, 140, 154, 155, 161, 162, 165, 168, 204, 232, 241, 244, **261**
haws 200, 207, 231, 232
hawthorn berries, *see haws*
hawthorn blossom 161, 165, 166, 206
hawthorn brandy 235
Hazel 80, 98, 200, 204, 241
headdress, making 90, 108, 172
healing 35-38,
Heartsease 188, 229
heart tonic herbs 258, 261, 264, 270, 276
Heather 210, 244
herbal baths 52, 101
herbal honeys, making **51**, 188, 233
herbal and flower syrups, making **163**, 232
herbs, drying **42**, 43, 162, 185
herbs, harvesting **41**, 115, 158, 180, 181, 184
herb journal 40
herbal oils **53**, 139, 148, 163, 186
herbs **40-53**
herb pillow, making 206
herbs, roots 82
herb suppliers 283
herb teas **43**, 45, 161
Holly 80, 107, 204, 241
holly touchwood, making 109
honey 51, 101, 120, 206
honey elixirs, *see elixirs*
honeys, herbal, *see herbal honeys*
Hops 49, 50, 102, 130, 132, 139, 140, 155, 209,243, **262**
hop beer 209
Humulus lupulus **262**
Hypericum perforatum **275**

incense from native plants, making 242
Imbolc 54, 58, 112, **122-125**
Imbolc doll or Earth spirit, making 125
immune system 50, 100
immune system herbs 253, 259, 270, 271
infused oils, *see herbal oils*

infusion or tisane 44
insight stones, making 125
insecticide, insect bites 253, 259, 265
insomnia, herbs 256, 277
iron tonic elixir 50
iron tonic herbs 252, 268

Jack by the Hedge, *see Garlic Mustard*
January into February 111-125
joint pains, herbs 258, 262, 275
journals, making 40, 113
June into July 175-193
July into August 195-217
Juniper 244

kidney tonic herbs 251, 253, 258, 270, 277
Kitchen Medicine **35-53**, 82-85, 100-103, 119-121, 136-144, 161-169, 184-188, 205-210, 230-237

labyrinth making 172
Lady's Mantle 50, 138, 139, 162, 202, 226, **263**
Lady's Smock 50, 132, 139, 140, 161, 162, 226, 229, **264**
Lammas 54, 58, 211-217
land 5-19, 74-77, 94-96, 112-114, 128-131, 152-160, 176-180, 196-200, 220-223
Lavender 49, 102, 139, 206, 244
lavender oil 187
lawns, productive 228
leaf mould 81
leaf tinctures, *see tinctures, leaf*
Lemon Balm 50, 139, 163
libations and offerings 199
Lime leaves 167, 168
liquid fertilisers, making 182
liver tonic herbs 229, 251, 258, 262, 273, 275, 277
Lughnasadh, *see Lammas*
lungs, herbs 251, 258, 265, 267
lymphatic tonic herbs 253, 267, 269

macerations, *see herbal oils*
Malus sylvestris **257**
Malva sylvestris **265**
Mallow, common 155, 188, **265**
Mallow oil 186
map making 197
March into April 127-149
Marigold (Calendula) oil 187
mask, making 90, 172

medicine bundle, making 192
medicine bag, making 192, 43
Meadowsweet 243
menopause elixir, 50
menopause, herbs 262, 263, 277
Mentha aquatica **266**
Mentha arvensis **266**
Mentha rotundifolia **266**
middles of celebrations 62
mindfulness 11,
Mint 50, 102, 121, 138, 139, 155, 162, 163, 188, **266**
moon, the 13, 58
mouthwash herbs 265, 266, 273
Mugwort 217, 243
Mullein 101, 120, 155, 206, 217, **267**
mullein flower oil 186

Native bulbs **226**, 230
native plants 17, 22, 23, 26–28, 36, 40
native pond plants 117
native trees, see trees
native wild flowers, see wild flowers
nerve tonic herbs 250, 256, 261, 262, 267, 269, 275, 276, 277
nest, making 147
Nettle 50, 101, 102, 115, 119, 121, 138, 139, 140, 142, 155, **268**
nettle and chickweed pesto 142
nettle soup 142
night walking 129, 220

Oak 155, 167, 177, 204, 241
October into November 73-91
opening circles 61
outside celebrations 63
oils, infused, see herbal oils

pain relief, herbs 265, 275, 276, 278
painting, see drawing and painting
perennials 249
pick-me-up elixir 50
pilgrimage 15, 145, 176
Pine 244
plants, growing natives 23-29, 158
plant-pot clusters 159
planting out 159
plants, transplanting 226
pond, making a 116
pond plants, native 117
Primrose 132, 161, 165, 201
primrose, growing 202
Primula veris **256**
Prunella vulgaris **273**

quarter festivals, the 57

Ramsons, see Garlic, Wild
Red Clover 50, 120, 139, 155, 161, 163, 165, 188, 229, **269**
restorative herbs 250, 259, 269, 273, 275, 277
Ribbed Plantain or Ribwort 101, 120
roots, digging up and drying 82
roots, dividing 226
root drinks 83,
root tinctures 82
Rosa canina **270**
rosehips 50, 120, 200, 207, 231, 232, 233, 244
rose oil 186
rose petals 121, 149, 163, 166, 188, 244
rose petal oil 149
Rosemary 50, 102, 121, 139, 163, 217, 244
Rose, wild 49, 50, 102, 244, **270**
Rowan 155, 200, 204, 207, 231, 241, 244, **271**
rowanberry jelly, making 235
Rumex acetosa **274**

Sage 50, 217, 244
Salad Burnet 132, 140, 142, 155, 201, 225, 229, **272**
Sambucus nigra **259**
Samhain 54, 58, 74, 86-91
sanctuary 22,
Sanguisorba minor **272**
seasonal celebrations 55- 67, 86-91, 103-109, 122-125, 144-149, 169-173
seed, collecting 201, 222, 225
seeds, inner 106, 124, 128, 144, 146
seeds, sowing 26, 132, 136, 147, 225
seed bombs 137
Self Heal 50, 229, **273**
Self Heal oil 186
September into October 219-244
Silver Birch, see Birch
skin, herbs 251, 253, 256, 257, 258, 259, 277
sleep herbs 50, 250, 259, 261, 262, 269, 276
sleep pillow 206
sloes 77, 84, 85,
sloe gin, making 84
sloe wine making 85
smudge stick, making 217

Solstices, the 57
solstice bush, making 108
Sorbus aucuparia **271**
sore throat, herbs 229, 259, 265, 267, 270, 273
Sorrel 115, 132, 140, 142, 155, 226, 229, **274**
sprains, herbs 250, 254, 265
Spring, On the Edge of 111-125
Spring 127-149
Spring Equinox 54, 57, 128, 144-149
spring greens 114
spring green pickle 121
storing herbs 43
springs and wells 153
spring tonics 119, 138
spring tonic herbs 251, 253, 255, 259, 264, 268
St John's Wort 50, 102, 121, 148, **275**
St John's Wort oil 148, 186
Stachys officinalis **250**
Stellaria media **251**
Summer, On the Edge of 150-173
Summer 175-93
Summer Solstice 54, 57, 176, 189-193
sunrise/sunset 12
Symphytum officinale **254**
syrups, making 163

talking stick, making 240-242
Taraxacum officinale **258**
tea bags, making 205
thresholds, natural 64, 94
Thyme 50, 101, 102, 139, 217, 244
tinctures, dosage 45
tinctures, flowers 162, 185
tinctures, fruit 231
tinctures, leaf 138, 162
tinctures, making **46**, 120, 185
tinctures, roots, 82
tisane 44
trees, 15, 95, 177, 203, 204
tree care 136
trees, creating living tree sculptures 98
tree leaf wines, making 167
tree planting 76, 97, 98, 203
trees, growing in pots 79
trees, growing from cuttings 80
tree seeds, collecting 222
trees, growing from seeds 204
trees, wild salads 168
Trifolium pratense **269**

Urtica dioica **268**

Valerian 49, 82, **276**
Valeriana officinalis **276**
Valerianella locusta **255**
Verbascum thapsus **267**
Verbena officinalis **277**
Vervain 49, 50, 102, 119, 121, 139, 188, **277**
vinegars, making 164
vinegars, flower
vinegars, fruit 209
Viola odorata **278**
Viola riviniana **278**
Violet 101, 102, 132, 161, 165, 188, 201, **278**
violets, growing 202
viral infections, herbs 253, 258, 270, 273, 275
vision quest 15, 145
visioning the future 106
vital energy, restoring 120

walking 4, 6, 14, 25, 74, 95, 104, 112, 123, 128, 129, 130, 145, 220
walking stick, making 215
wild flowers, growing 133-136
wildlife garden, making a 116
Willow 80, 98, 108, 241
wine, flowers, making 166
wine, fruit, making 207
wine, tree leaf, making 167
Wintercress 115, 132, 140, 201, 202, 225, **279**
Winter, On the Edge of 73-91
Winter 93-109
winter greens, sowing 225
winter salad plants 202
Winter Solstice 54, 57, 94, 103-109
Wood Sorrel 114, 115, 132
wonder wander 15, 145
Wormwood 217
wound herbs 250, 257, 259, 261, 267, 273, 275, 277, 280

Yarrow 50, 102, 119, 155, 162, 226, 230, **280**
Yarrow oil 163

ABOUT GLENNIE KINDRED

Glennie Kindred is the author of eleven books on Earth wisdom, native plants and trees and celebrating the Earth's cycles. She has a strong and committed following and enjoys sharing her insights through a wide range of popular workshops and talks. She is renowned for her ability to enthuse people with inspiration to engage with the natural environment and the power that we can individually and collectively create to bring about positive change, both for ourselves and for the Earth.

She lives in a small market town in Derbyshire with her partner Brian Boothby, where she enjoys gardening, kitchen medicine, many creative projects, her friends and family, and her local community. She is active in the transition towns initiative. Her passions include walking the land barefoot, guerrilla gardening, travelling, and being alive to the wonders and delights of the natural world. She has three children, May, Jack and Jerry and a granddaughter, Evie Rose.

OTHER BOOKS BY GLENNIE KINDRED

Earth Cycles of Celebration, published by Glennie Kindred 1991, revised 2002

Sacred Tree, published by Glennie Kindred 1995, revised 2003

Tree Ogham, published by Glennie Kindred 1997

Creating Ceremony (with Lu Garner), published by Glennie Kindred 2002

Elements of Change, published by Glennie Kindred 2009

Hedgerow Cookbook, published by Wooden Books 1999, revised 2002

Herbal Healers, published by Wooden Books 1999, revised 2002

Earth Wisdom, published by Hay House 2004, revised 2011

Earth Alchemy (formally Alchemist's Journey), published by Hay House 2005, revised 2013

Sacred Celebrations, first published 2001. Revised and re-published Spring 2014

For signed copies of all publications, monthly native plants and trees updates, courses, talks and workshops, prints and cards

www.glenniekindred.co.uk

Inspiration for
Sustainable Living

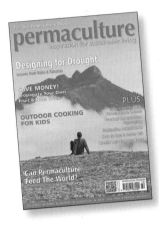

Permaculture is a magazine that helps you transform your home, garden and community, and save money.

Permaculture magazine offers tried and tested ways of creating flexible, low cost approaches to sustainable living, helping you to:

- Make informed ethical choices
- Grow and source organic food
- Put more into your local community
- Build energy efficiency into your home
- Find courses, contacts and opportunities
- Live in harmony with people and the planet

Permaculture magazine is published quarterly for enquiring minds and original thinkers everywhere. Each issue gives you practical, thought provoking articles written by leading experts as well as fantastic ecofriendly tips from readers!

permaculture, ecovillages, ecobuilding, organic gardening, agroforestry, sustainable agriculture, appropriate technology, downshifting, community development, human-scale economy ... and much more!

Permaculture magazine gives you access to a unique network of people and introduces you to pioneering projects in Britain and around the world. Subscribe today and start enriching your life without overburdening the planet!

PERMANENT PUBLICATIONS
The Sustainability Centre, East Meon, Hampshire GU32 1HR, UK
Tel: 01730 823 311 Fax: 01730 823 322   (Overseas: int code +44-1730)
Email: info@permaculture.co.uk

To subscribe and for daily updates, vist our exciting and dynamic website:
www.permaculture.co.uk

More books from Permanent Publications

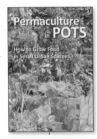
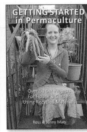
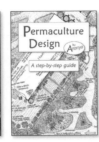
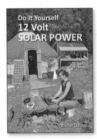
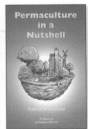
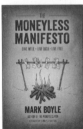
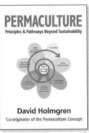
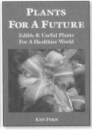
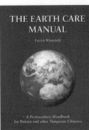
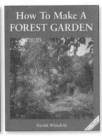
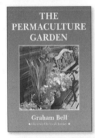
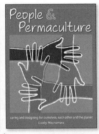
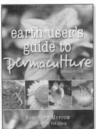
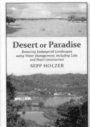
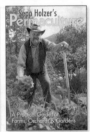
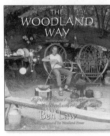
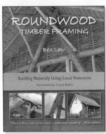
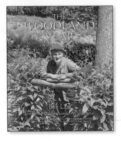
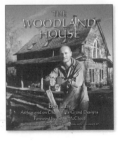